Advanced Signal Processing on Brain Event-Related Potentials

Filtering ERPs in Time, Frequency and Space Domains Sequentially and Simultaneously

Advanced Signal Processing on Brain Event-Related Potentials

Filtering ERPs in Time, Frequency and Space Domains Sequentially and Simultaneously

Fengyu Cong
Dalian University of Technology, China

Tapani Ristaniemi
University of Jyväskylä, Finland

Heikki Lyytinen
University of Jyväskylä, Finland

World Scientific

NEW JERSEY · LONDON · SINGAPORE · BEIJING · SHANGHAI · HONG KONG · TAIPEI · CHENNAI

Published by

World Scientific Publishing Co. Pte. Ltd.
5 Toh Tuck Link, Singapore 596224
USA office: 27 Warren Street, Suite 401-402, Hackensack, NJ 07601
UK office: 57 Shelton Street, Covent Garden, London WC2H 9HE

British Library Cataloguing-in-Publication Data
A catalogue record for this book is available from the British Library.

ADVANCED SIGNAL PROCESSING ON BRAIN EVENT-RELATED POTENTIALS
Filtering ERPs in Time, Frequency and Space Domains Sequentially and Simultaneously

ISBN 978-981-4623-08-7

Typeset by Stallion Press
Email: enquiries@stallionpress.com

Contents

Preface   xv

List of Abbreviations   xx

Chapter 1   Introduction   1

  1.1   Motivation   1
       1.1.1   Categories of EEG data   1
       1.1.2   Signal processing of EEG data   2
  1.2   Example of Conventional ERP Data Processing   3
  1.3   Linear Transform Model of ERP Data   5
  1.4   Existing Problems in Conventional ERP Data
       Processing and Their Solutions   7
       1.4.1   Assumptions for the averaging step   7
       1.4.2   Problems in the assumptions of the averaging
             step   7
       1.4.3   Solutions   9
  1.5   ERP Data for the Demonstration in This Book   10
  References   10

Chapter 2   Wavelet Filter Design Based on Frequency
Responses for Filtering ERP Data With Duration
of One Epoch   15

  2.1   Correlation   15
  2.2   Impulse Response and Frequency Response   16
  2.3   Moving-Average Model-Based FIR Digital Filter   18
       2.3.1   Interpreting the digital filter in terms
             of correlation   18

2.3.2   Problems of the digital filter in removing artifacts
         and their solutions   18
2.4   DFT-Based Digital Filter   20
      2.4.1   Definition of DFT   20
      2.4.2   Interpreting DFT using correlation   20
      2.4.3   DFT-based digital filter   21
      2.4.4   Problems of the DFT filter and their corresponding
               solutions   23
2.5   Wavelet Transform   24
      2.5.1   Definition of wavelet transform   24
      2.5.2   Interpreting the wavelet transform using
               correlation   25
      2.5.3   Differences between the Fourier
               and wavelet transforms   25
      2.5.4   Implementation of DWT   26
2.6   Wavelet Filter Design Based on Frequency Response . . .   27
      2.6.1   Introduction to wavelet filter   27
      2.6.2   Key issues in the wavelet filter design   28
      2.6.3   Determination of the number of levels   28
               2.6.3.1 Existing problem and current solution   . .   28
               2.6.3.2 New solution   28
      2.6.4   Frequency division at different DWT levels:
               Overlapped frequency contents at different
               levels   29
      2.6.5   Frequency division in the first level of DWT:
               The cutoff frequency of the LP and HP filters is
               $Fs/2$ instead of $Fs/4$ 31
      2.6.6   Selection of the detail coefficients at some levels for
               signal reconstruction   31
               2.6.6.1 Existing problem and current solution   . .   31
               2.6.6.2 New solution   33
      2.6.7   Choosing the wavelet for the wavelet filter in ERP
               studies   33
               2.6.7.1 Existing problem and current solution   . .   33
               2.6.7.2 New solution   33

2.6.8   Effect of sampling frequency
on the wavelet filter 36

2.7   Linear Superposition Rule of the Wavelet Filter
and Benefit of the Wavelet Filter in Contrast
to the Digital Filter 37

2.8   Comparison Between the Wavelet and Digital Filters: Case
Study on the Waveform and Magnitude Spectrum 39

2.9   Recommendation for the Wavelet Filter Design 41

2.10 Summary: ERP Data Processing Approach Using DFT or
Wavelet Filter 41

2.11 Existing Key Problem and Potential Solution 42

2.12 MATLAB Codes 42

2.12.1 DFT filter function 42

2.12.2 Wavelet filter function 43

2.12.3 Frequency responses of DFT filter
and wavelet filter 44

References 48

**Chapter 3   Individual-Level ICA to Extract the ERP
Components from the Averaged EEG Data**   **51**

3.1   Classic ICA Theory 51

3.1.1 Brief history 51

3.1.2 ICA model, assumptions, and solution in obtaining
independent components 52

3.1.2.1 Model 52

3.1.2.2 Classification of the ICA models 54

3.1.2.3 Assumptions 54

3.1.2.4 Solution 54

3.1.3 ICA algorithm and indeterminacies of independent
components 55

3.1.3.1 Classification of ICA algorithms based on
the ICA models 55

3.1.3.2 ICA algorithm for the determined
model 55

3.1.3.3 Implementation of the ICA algorithm . . . 56

3.1.3.4 Definitions of the global and local
optimization of ICA 56
3.1.3.5 Indeterminacies of the independent
components 57
3.2 ICA Theory in ERP Data Processing: Back Projection . . . 58
3.2.1 Reconsideration of the linear transform
model of EEG 60
3.2.2 Back-projection of an ICA component to correct the
indeterminacies in the variance and polarity 65
3.2.2.1 Introduction to back-projection 65
3.2.2.2 Back-projection under global
optimization 66
3.2.2.3 Back-projection under local
optimization 71
3.3 Indeterminacies and Determinacies of ICA on EEG 73
3.3.1 Indeterminacies of ICA on EEG 78
3.3.2 Determinacies in ICA on EEG 78
3.3.3 Obtaining the determinacies of ICA
on EEG in practice 78
3.4 Practical Consideration of the ICA Model of EEG 79
3.4.1 Noisy or noise-free ICA models 79
3.4.2 Can correcting artifacts and extracting the ERP
components be realized simultaneously? 80
3.4.3 Group- or individual-level ICA 81
3.4.4 Converting the over-determined model to the
determined model 82
3.4.5 Converting the under-determined model to the
determined model 83
3.5 MOS to Determine the Number of Sources 83
3.5.1 Introduction to MOS 83
3.5.2 Theoretical eigenvalues and MOS 84
3.5.3 MOS in practice 85
3.5.3.1 Information-theory-based methods 85
3.5.3.2 SORTE 86
3.5.3.3 RAE 87
3.5.3.4 Simulation for MOS 87

3.6   Key Practical Issues for ICA to Extract the ERP
        Components   91
        3.6.1   Are the concatenated single-trial or averaged EEG
                 data better for ICA to extract the ERP components
                 under the assumption of independence?   91
        3.6.2   Number of samples and number of sources   92
        3.6.3   Reducing the number of sources in averaged EEG
                 data and increasing the SNR   92
                 3.6.3.1   Filtering the averaged EEG data   92
                 3.6.3.2   Appropriately designed wavelet filter . . .   93
        3.6.4   Validation of the stability of ICA
                 decomposition   95
3.7   Systematic ICA Approach on the Extraction of ERP
        Components from Averaged EEG Data (Responses of
        Stimuli) Collected by a High-Density Array   97
        3.7.1   Ordinary ERP data: Ordinarily averaged
                 EEG data over single trials of one stimulus
                 and one subject   97
        3.7.2   Wavelet filtering of averaged EEG data   99
        3.7.3   Converting the over-determined model to the
                 determined model: Dimension reduction   99
        3.7.4   ICA decomposition and stability analysis   101
        3.7.5   Selection of the components of interest   107
        3.7.6   Back-projection of selected components   107
3.8   Systematic ICA Approach to Extract the ERP Components
        from the Averaged EEG Data (DW) Collected by
        Low-Density Array   107
        3.8.1   Motivation   107
        3.8.2   Introduction to DW   108
        3.8.3   Six steps of the systematic ICA approach to extract
                 the MMN component from the DW   108
3.9   Reliability of the Independent Components Extracted by the
        Systematic ICA Approach from Averaged EEG Data   . . .   114
        3.9.1   Simulation study: Sufficiency of several
                 hundreds of samples in extracting a few
                 dozens of sources   114

3.9.2   Are bump-like independent components reasonable
when the systematic ICA approach is applied on the
averaged EEG data?   116

3.10 Benefits of the Wavelet Filter in the Systematic ICA
Approach to Extract the ERP Components from Averaged
EEG Data   117

3.11 Relationship among the Global Optimization
of the ICA Decomposition, Stability of the ICA
Decomposition, ICA Algorithm, and Number
of Extracted Components   118

3.12 Summary   119

3.13 Existing Key Problems and Potential Solutions   120

3.14 MATLAB Codes   121

3.14.1 Systematic ICA approach on averaged EEG data
collected by high-density array   121

3.14.2 Model order selection   123

3.14.3 Systematic ICA approach on averaged EEG data
collected by low-density array   124

References   124

**Chapter 4   Multi-Domain Feature of the ERP Extracted
by NTF: New Approach for Group-Level Analysis of ERPs**   131

4.1   TFR of ERPs and High-Order Tensor   131

4.1.1   TFR of ERPs: Evoked and induced brain activity .   131

4.1.1.1   Difference in the TFR of an ERP
between the evoked and induced
brain activities   132

4.1.1.2   TFR of an ERP used in this study: TFR of
the averaged EEG   132

4.1.1.3   ROI of the TFR of the ERP   133

4.1.2   High-order ERP tensor   134

4.1.2.1   ERP waveform tensors   134

4.1.2.2   ERP tensors of TFRs of averaged
EEG data   134

4.2   Introduction of the Tensor Decomposition   135

4.2.1   Brief history   135

4.2.2   Basis for tensor decomposition 136

      4.2.2.1   Inner and outer products 136

      4.2.2.2   Outer product of multiple vectors 137

      4.2.2.3   Mode-n tensor matrix product 137

4.2.3   CPD model 137

      4.2.3.1   Simple illustration of the CPD 137

      4.2.3.2   General definition of CPD 138

      4.2.3.3   Uniqueness analysis of CPD 138

      4.2.3.4   Difference between matrix decomposition
                  and CPD 139

4.2.4   Tucker decomposition model 139

4.2.5   Difference between the CPD and Tucker
         decomposition models 140

4.2.6   Fit of a tensor decomposition model 141

4.2.7   Classic algorithms of the CPD and Tucker
         decomposition 142

4.2.8   NTF 143

4.2.9   Why is a nonnegative ERP tensor of the TFR used
         instead of an ERP tensor of a waveform? 143

4.3   Multi-Domain Feature of ERP 144

4.3.1   Conventional features of an ERP (averaged EEG)
         versus features of spontaneous and single-trial
         EEGs 144

      4.3.1.1   Conventional features of an ERP (averaged
                  EEG) 144

      4.3.1.2   Features of spontaneous and single-trial
                  EEGs for pattern recognition 145

      4.3.1.3   Difference between the conventional
                  features of an ERP for cognitive
                  neuroscience and the features of
                  spontaneous and single-trial EEGs for
                  pattern recognition 145

4.3.2   Brief review of the EEG data analysis by tensor
         decomposition 146

4.3.3   Multi-domain feature of ERPs extracted by NCPD
         from the fourth-order ERP tensor of TFRs 147

4.3.3.1 Feature extraction 147

4.3.3.2 Feature selection 149

4.3.3.3 Group-level analysis of the multi-domain feature of an ERP 150

4.3.3.4 Drawback in using the fourth-order ERP tensor of TFRs 152

4.3.4 Multi-domain feature of ERPs extracted by NCPD from a third-order ERP tensor of the TFRs 153

4.3.5 Multi-domain feature of an ERP extracted by NTD 154

4.3.6 Third-order ERP tensor of the TFRs for NTF . . . 159

4.3.6.1 ERP tensor of the TFRs for individual topographies 159

4.3.6.2 ERP tensor of the TFRs for individual temporal components 159

4.3.6.3 ERP tensor of the TFRs for individual spectra 159

4.3.7 Uniqueness analysis 159

4.4 Adaptive and Objective Extraction of ROI from the TFRs of the ERPs 160

4.5 Key Issues in Using the NTF to Extract the Multi-Domain Feature of an ERP from the ERP Tensor of the TFRs 160

4.5.1 LRA-based fast NTF algorithm 160

4.5.2 Determining the number of extracted components 161

4.5.2.1 MOS 162

4.5.2.2 ARD 162

4.5.2.3 Data-driven methods 163

4.5.3 Stability of the multi-domain feature of the ERP extracted by the NTF 164

4.5.4 How many components can be appropriately extracted by the NTF with knowledge of ERPs taken into account? 166

4.5.5 Which tensor decomposition model should be chosen for the NTF? 167

4.6 Summary 168
4.7 Existing Key Problem and Potential Solution 171
4.8 MATLAB Codes 171
References 172

Chapter 5 Analysis of Ongoing EEG by NTF During Real-World Music Experiences 179

5.1 Motivation 179
5.2 Third-Order Ongoing EEG Tensor of a Spectrogram 180
5.3 Musical Features of the Naturalistic Music 181
5.4 NTF on the Spectrogram of Ongoing EEG 183
5.5 Summary 187
5.6 Existing Problem and Solution 187
References 187

Appendix Introduction to Basic Knowledge of Mismatch Negativity 191

A.1 Brief History of MMN 191
A.2 Paradigm to Elicit MMN 192
A.3 Basic Psychological Knowledge of MMN 195
A.4 Properties of MMN 195
    A.4.1 Temporal property 196
    A.4.2 Spectral property 196
    A.4.3 Time-frequency property 197
    A.4.4 Topography 199
References 200

Preface

The brain event-related potential (ERP) has been an extensively used tool for cognitive neuroscience. For example, in order to elicit a very interesting and an important ERP component, mismatch negativity (MMN) invented by Risto Näätänen, a sequence of short auditory stimuli (standard, e.g., 200 ms) is presented interspersing in the sequence randomly a different (deviant) sound infrequently at least tens but often hundreds of times with short (e.g., 300 ms) intervals between the sounds. Such an ERP component, i.e., an aspect of interest in the electroencephalography (EEG) waveform which reflects activity of the brain, is measurable nonintrusively from the surface of the head. It is extracted by averaging post-stimulus segments of EEG from certain surface locations typically for a length of 300–1000 ms separately for each of such repeated stimuli. In the case of MMN, the computational manipulation of the averages of responses to the mentioned two stimulus types continues to define their difference to learn how the brain notifies the change in the auditory world. The traditional way to do so has been to simply compute a difference waveform between these two averages.

Before the averaging, preprocessing continuous EEG data (before segmentation according to the stimulus sequence) or concatenated single-trial EEG data (after segmentation according to the stimulus sequence) is necessary for rejecting and/or correcting artifacts. Therefore, the data preprocessing methods are often applied on the very long EEG data, for example, independent component analysis (ICA). As for the averaged EEG data, signal processing methods except the averaging have been seldom applied in the existing research literature to extract ERP components. One critical issue is that the number of samples in the averaged EEG data is often very limited, which probably results in overfitting for signal processing. Everything has the dark side and the bright side. In the averaged EEG, signal-to-noise ratio (SNR) is much higher than that in the continuous EEG, or the concatenated single-trial EEG, or the single-trial EEG. The higher SNR is, the better results signal processing methods may produce. Inspired by these issues, in this book, we introduce our research of ERP data processing, i.e., how to develop and apply advanced signal processing methods to extract ERP components from the averaged EEG in an ERP experiment for individual subjects and for group subjects.

Chapter 1 further defines the motivation to write the book, reviews conventional ERP data processing methods, states existing problems, and briefly presents solutions to the problems.

Chapter 2 introduces some basic knowledge for correlation, digital filter and Fourier transform, and also describes how to design an appropriate wavelet filter in terms of the frequency response of the filter. In this chapter, it is the first time that digital filter, Fourier transform, and wavelet transform are interpreted by correlation. We believe that it is easier for the readers who are not experienced in mathematics to understand concepts of digital filter, Fourier transform, and wavelet transform.

Chapter 3 is devoted to the design of a systematic ICA approach including six steps to extract ERPs' components from the averaged EEG data of one subject and one experimental condition. With the new approach applied, the ERP data are indeed filtered in the time, frequency, and space domains sequentially. Particularly, we introduce why and how the variance and the polarity of an independent component can be corrected in theory and practice and how to estimate the number of components to be extracted by ICA.

Chapter 4 introduces a new biomarker of ERP for group-level analysis. It is the multi-domain feature of an ERP extracted by tensor decomposition with nonnegative constraints from time-frequency representations (TFRs) of the averaged EEG. It should be noted that the TFR of ERP data is usually in terms of absolute value of wavelet transform, and values of TFRs are nonnegative. Time-frequency analysis has been very popular for analysis of ERPs and it can be used for both the single-trial EEG data and the averaged EEG data. When the averaged EEG data are transformed into the time-frequency domain, the data of multiple channels and multiple subjects become multi-way. A multi-way data array is named as a "tensor" in mathematics. The high-order ERP tensor of TFRs of the averaged EEG includes multiple modes of time, frequency, space, and subject. Therefore, the nonnegative tensor factorization (one category of tensor decomposition methods) can be applied to decompose the ERP tensor of TFRs into the temporal, spectral, and spatial components, as well as the multi-domain features of ERPs. The advantage of the multi-domain feature of an ERP is that it reveals the strength of brain activity in light of its properties in the time, frequency, and space domains simultaneously. In terms of different ways to organize an ERP tensor of TFRs, multi-domain feature of an ERP allows examining individuals' ERP informatics in one domain and projecting individuals' ERP data to other domains which are common for individuals.

Chapter 5 describes our recent research about analysis of ongoing EEG when a participant listens to a piece of the naturalistic music stimulus. Indeed, ERPs are elicited by the short and rapidly repeated stimulus which seldom occurs in practice. Therefore, in order to know brain activity during real-world experiences, it is necessary to analyze brain data elicited by the long and nonrepeated stimulus, i.e., naturalistic stimulus. We use nonnegative tensor factorization to decompose a third-order ongoing EEG tensor of spectrogram into temporal components, spectral components, and spatial components. We try our best to succeed in finding brain activity elicited by the music stimulus.

In this book, many examples are taken for illustration of the advanced signal processing methods. They are based on the ERP data of MMN. Therefore, in the Appendix, we introduce basic knowledge of MMN, which assists to understand the contents of the book. Furthermore, MATLAB codes and demo ERP data are provided for reference via http://www.escience.cn/people/cong/index.html.

Contributions to the book are as the following: From 2007 to 2012, Cong, Ristaniemi, and Lyytinen had over 100 times' discussion for most of the contents of the book. Cong came up with the ideas of the wavelet filter, the systematic ICA approach, and the multi-domain feature of an ERP. Ristaniemi assisted to trim the ideas. Lyytinen supervised the interpretation of advance signal processing results in terms of user knowledge of an experienced researcher who has been using ERP-recordings for learning to understand human mind. Cong wrote the proposal of the book and Ristaniemi revised it. Cong wrote the whole book and Lyytinen revised the preface, Chapter 1, and the appendix.

We thank Professor Paavo Leppänen, Dr. Piia Astikainen, Dr. Jarmo Hämäläinen, Professor Petri Toiviainen, and Dr. Jukka Kaartinen in the University of Jyväskylä; Professor Jari Hietanen in the University of Tampere; Dr. Minna Huotilainen in the University of Helsinki in Finland; Professor Andrzej Cichocki, Dr. Qibin Zhao, Dr. Guoxu Zhou, and Dr. Anh-Huy Phan in RIKEN Brain Science Institute in Japan; Dr. Qiang Wu in the Shandong University; and Professor Hua Shu, Dr. Hong Li, and Dr. Youyi Liu in the Beijing Normal University in China; and Dr. Nicole Landi in Haskins Laboratories in the Yale University in USA, for providing their demo ERP data and discussions on the ERP data processing. Particularly, Cong thanks Professor TianShuang Qiu in Dalian University of Technology in China for providing the excellent working environment to write the book. Cong thanks Mz Qian Zhao (Dalian Development Zone, Dalian, China) for helping to proofread the book and her moral support in writing the book. Cong also thanks the financial support from TEKES in Finland (MIPCOM and MUSCLES projects), the Fundamental Research Funds for the Central Universities [DUT14RC(3)037], and for XingHai Scholar in Dalian University of Technology in China, and National Natural Science Foundation of China (Grant No. 81471742).

This monograph includes knowledge of ERPs, basic signal processing methods (e.g., digital filter and Fourier transform), and advanced signal processing methods (e.g., wavelet transform, ICA, and tensor decomposition). Therefore, it can be used as a reference for senior undergraduate students, postgraduate students, and researchers in the relevant fields both as a research book and as a textbook.

During the writing of the book in the spring of 2014, Tapani was sick. We hope that Tapani recovers completely as soon as possible!

Professor Fengyu Cong at Dalian in China

Department of Biomedical Engineering, Faculty of Electronic Information and Electrical Engineering, Dalian University of Technology, China, and Department of Mathematical Information Technology, University of Jyväskylä, Finland

Email: cong@dlut.edu.cn

Homepage: http://www.escience.cn/people/cong/index.html

Professor Tapani Ristaniemi at Jyväskylä in Finland

Department of Mathematical Information Technology, University of Jyväskylä, Finland

Email: tapani.ristaniemi@jyu.fi

Homepage: http://users.jyu.fi/~riesta/

Professor Heikki Lyytinen at Jyväskylä in Finland

Department of Psychology, University of Jyväskylä, Finland

Email: heikki.j.lyytinen@jyu.fi

Homepage: http://users.jyu.fi/~hlyytine/

January 2015

List of Abbreviations

AD	—	Attention Deficit
ADHD	—	Attention Deficit Hyperactivity Disorder
AIC	—	Akaike's Information Criterion
ALS	—	Alternating Least Square
ANOVA	—	Analysis of Variance
ARD	—	Automatic Relevance Determination
BCI	—	Brain–Computer Interface
BSS	—	Blind Source Separation
CP	—	Canonical Polyadic
CPD	—	Canonical Polyadic Decomposition
CWT	—	Continuous Waveform Transform
DFT	—	Discrete Fourier Transform
DW	—	Difference Wave
DWT	—	Discrete Wavelet Transform
EEG	—	Electroencephalography
ERP	—	Event-Related Potential
FIR	—	Finite Impulse Response
fMRI	—	Functional Magnetic Resonance Imaging
HALS	—	Hierarchical ALS
HP	—	High-Pass
ICA	—	Independent Component Analysis
IIR	—	Infinite Impulse Response
ISI	—	Inter-Stimulus-Interval
KIC	—	Kullback–Leibler Information Criterion
LP	—	Low-Pass
LRA	—	Low-Rank Approximation

LRANMF	—	LRA-Based NMF
MDL	—	Minimum Description Length
MEG	—	Magnetoencephalography
MMN	—	Mismatch Negativity
MOS	—	Model Order Selection
NCPD	—	Nonnegative Canonical Polyadic Decomposition
NMF	—	Nonnegative Matrix Factorization
NTF	—	Nonnegative Tensor Factorization
NTD	—	Nonnegative Tucker Decomposition
PARAFAC	—	Parallel Factor Analysis
PCA	—	Principal Component Analysis
RAE	—	Ratio of Adjacent Eigenvalues
RD	—	Reading Disability
ROI	—	Region of Interest
SNR	—	Signal-to-Noise Ratio
SOA	—	Stimulus-Onset-Asynchrony
SoNR	—	Source-to-Noise Ratio
SORTE	—	Second ORder sTatistic of the Eigenvalues
TFR	—	Time-Frequency Representation
vMMN	—	Visual MMN

Chapter 1

Introduction

In this chapter, we introduce our motivation for writing this book, review conventional event-related potential (ERP) data processing methods, state the existing problems, and briefly present solutions to these problems.

1.1 Motivation

1.1.1 *Categories of EEG data*

Electrical activities in a human brain produced by the firing of neurons can be safely recorded through electrodes distributed over the scalp. Such recordings are termed as electroencephalography (EEG) (Niedermeyer & Lopes da Silva, 2004). EEG can be divided into three categories according to the different experimental paradigms.

The first paper to introduce EEG that described the spontaneous electrical activities/sources of the brain was written by a German psychiatrist — Professor Hans Berger — in 1929 (Berger, 1929). Since Professor Berger recorded EEG, spontaneous EEG has been used to discriminate brain activities between typical and clinical populations. For example, Berger also studied the diagnosis of epilepsy using spontaneous EEG. Currently, the clinical use of spontaneous EEG includes the diagnosis of coma, encephalopathy, brain death, tumors, strokes, and other focal brain disorders (Niedermeyer & Lopes da Silva, 2004). In experiments conducted to obtain the spontaneous EEG, no external stimuli were presented to the participants.

In everyday life, people often respond to many afferent stimuli, e.g., a sudden call, a flash of light, a changing image, and so on. Under these conditions, the brain activity is related to these events. Moreover, spontaneous EEG may include thousands of spontaneous brain processes, but the evoked/event-related responses in the brain to the outside stimuli might reflect a human thought or perception. The evoked/event-related response was first studied by the Davis couple between 1935 and 1936, who published their studies in 1939 (Davis, Davis, Loomis, Harvey, & Hobart, 1939). Today, ERPs elicited by controlled, short, and rapidly repeated stimuli are extensively used in brain science research (Luck, 2005). The use of ERPs is an effective method of studying the brain functions of the local region in the cortex.

Recently, ongoing EEG has been studied when a naturalistic, long, and nonrepeated stimulus (for example, music or film clip) is presented to the subjects (Cong, Alluri, *et al.*, 2013; Dmochowski, Sajda, Dias, & Parra, 2012). Using this naturalistic stimulus, the study of the brain functions during real-world experiences has been made possible.

1.1.2 *Signal processing of EEG data*

Spontaneous EEG and ERPs are extensively used in brain sciences and technologies, and ongoing EEG is a very new subject that is still under investigation from many perspectives. Regardless of what EEG type is studied, processing the EEG for artifact rejection and/or correction is necessary when EEG data collection is complete (Cong, Alluri, *et al.*, 2013; Luck, 2005; Niedermeyer & Lopes da Silva, 2004). Thereafter, data processing and analysis of the spontaneous activity can be straightforwardly done in spontaneous EEG experiments. However, in ERP (or ongoing EEG) experiments, the preprocessed EEG data are still a mixture of ERPs and spontaneous EEG (or ongoing and spontaneous EEGs). Therefore, to obtain the ERPs or ongoing EEG, the mixture must be separated using signal processing methods.

For clinical application of spontaneous EEGs and single-trial ERP data in a brain–computer interface (BCI), the data processing and analysis are mostly based on machine-learning methods, which include feature extraction, selection, and classification (Adeli & Ghosh-Dastidar, 2010;

Tan & Nijholt, 2010). ERPs are still primarily used in cognitive neuroscience. In most cases, the machine-learning methods for spontaneous EEGs are inappropriate for ERPs. Currently, excellent books are available that introduce the ERP mechanisms (Nunez & Srinivasan, 2005) and technologies (Luck, 2005), EEG signal processing for ERPs and spontaneous EEG (Sanei & Chambers, 2007).

Following the development of signal processing methods, wavelet filter (Quian Quiroga & Garcia, 2003), independent component analysis (ICA) (Onton, Westerfield, Townsend, & Makeig, 2006), and tensor decomposition (Morup, Hansen, & Arnfred, 2007) have been applied to extract ERPs. These three methods filter the ERPs in the time-frequency, time-space, and time-frequency-space domains, respectively. We found that some key problems arising from the use of the wavelet filter, ICA, and tensor decomposition in studying the ERPs have not been very well addressed, which motivated us to resolve these problems. After six years of research, we have come up with some solutions and decided to write this book to introduce our concept in using the wavelet filter, ICA, and tensor decomposition to extract the ERPs from preprocessed EEG data. We should note that EEG data preprocessing is not taken up in this book.

Advanced signal processing algorithms are typically based on complicated mathematics. To make this book much simpler for wider disciplines, we did not include the complicated mathematical algorithms of the wavelet filter, ICA, or tensor decomposition; however, their basic theories are presented. Moreover, to illustrate the basic theories, many examples (showing the ERP waveforms, spectra, topographies, and so on) are provided. Furthermore, to increase the utility of the wavelet filter, ICA, and tensor decomposition in extracting the ERPs, we also demonstrate the MATLAB (The Mathworks, Inc., Natick, MA, 2010) codes and ERP data.

1.2 Example of Conventional ERP Data Processing

ERPs are usually elicited by short and rapidly repeated stimuli. Figure 1.1 shows an example of the stimulus sequence of a passive oddball paradigm. The faces that represent happy and fearful emotions, which act as deviant stimuli, are much fewer than faces with neutral emotions, used as standard stimuli. Before the experiment, the participants choose some favorite

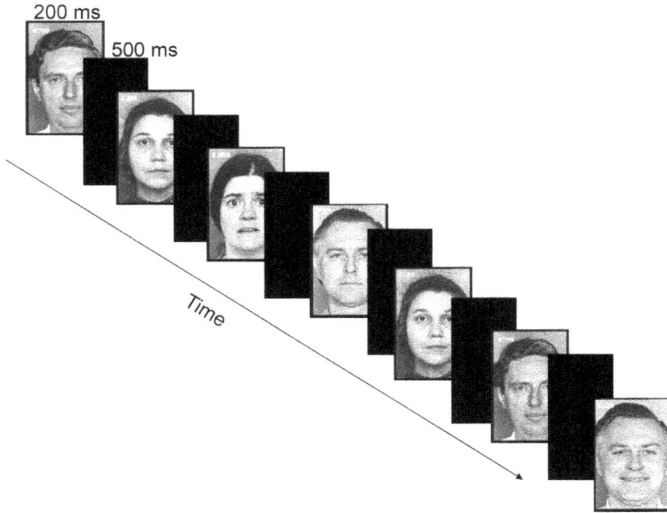

Figure 1.1 Example of ERP stimulus sequence.

auditory materials (e.g., speech or music). During the experiment, both visual stimuli and auditory materials are presented, and the participants are instructed to look at the faces shown in a computer screen and ignore the visual stimuli but pay attention to the auditory materials (thus, the paradigm is called "passive").

Figure 1.2 shows an example that introduces the whole data processing procedure of the ERP study (Talsma, 2008). During the experiment, continuous EEG data are recorded, as shown by the first row in Figure 1.2. Then, the continuous EEG data are segmented into single-trial EEG data according to the stimulus sequence. Subsequently, the single trials that include the artifacts are rejected. Next, the remaining single-trial EEG data for the same type of stimuli are averaged to produce the ERP waveforms, as shown at the bottom of Figure 1.2.

After the ERP waveforms are generated, the peak parameters of an ERP are measured, e.g., peak amplitude and peak latency. They are further used in the statistical analysis to draw some conclusions. Obviously, the artifact rejection and averaging steps are critical in the conventional ERP data processing.

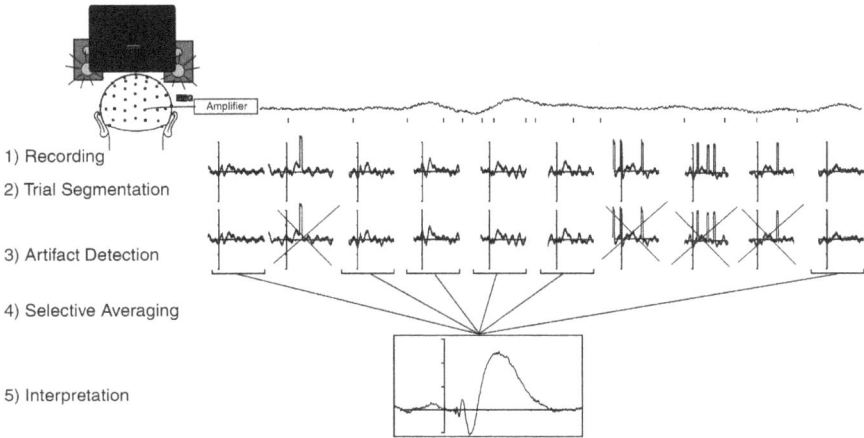

Figure 1.2 Example that introduces the whole ERP data processing procedure [adapted from Talsma (2008)].

Hereinafter, subsequent "ERP data" usages in this book indicates the averaged EEG over single trials. In the next section, we introduce the mathematical model of the ERP data.

1.3 Linear Transform Model of ERP Data

The EEG data can be represented by a linear transform model (Makeig, Jung, Bell, Ghahremani, & Sejnowski, 1997; Nunez & Srinivasan, 2005) as shown in Figure 1.3 (Jung *et al.*, 2000). In the brain cortex, many electrical sources exist. Each source includes two modes, namely, time and space. The spatial component does not change over time and reflects the spatial distribution over the scalp, and the temporal component reveals the time evolution. Each electrode along the scalp records the mixture of the scaled versions of the temporal components of the many sources, which is how the linear transform model is formulated. We should note that the absolute value of the scale is smaller than one because of volume conduction (Nunez & Srinivasan, 2005).

Next, we consider an example of the EEG data in an ERP experiment for mathematical illustration of the EEG data model. The single-trial EEG

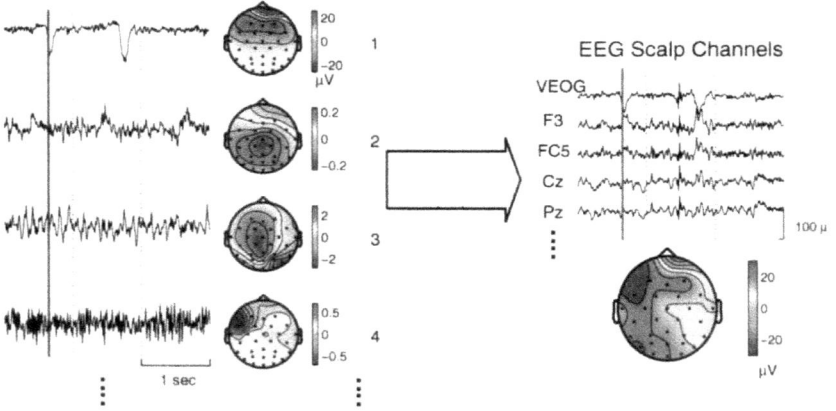

Figure 1.3   Example of EEG model [adapted from Jung *et al.* (2000)].

data (free of artifacts) in the experiment can be modeled as follows:

$$z_m(t, \ell) = \alpha_{m,1}(\ell) \cdot s_1(t, \ell) + \alpha_{m,2}(\ell) \cdot s_2(t, \ell) + \cdots + \alpha_{m,n}(\ell)$$
$$\cdot s_n(t, \ell) + \cdots + \alpha_{m,N(\ell)}(\ell) \cdot s_N(t, \ell) + v_m(t, \ell) \qquad (1\text{-}1)$$

where

m is the number of the sensor/the electrode here; $m = 1, 2, \ldots, M$;

t is the number of the sample; and $t = 1, 2, \ldots, T$;

l is the number of the single trial; $l = 1, 2, \ldots, L$;

n is the number of the electrical source; $n = 1, 2, \ldots, N(l)$;

$z_m(t, \ell)$ denotes the recorded EEG data;

$s_n(t, \ell)$ represents the electrical source, and it can be a stimulus-elicited or a spontaneous brain activity;

$\alpha_{m,n}(\ell)$ is the coefficient between source #n and the point where electrode #m is placed along the scalp; and

$v_m(t, \ell)$ denotes the sensor noise.

After the averaging, the ERP data can be expressed as

$$z_m(t) = \frac{1}{L} \sum_{l=1}^{L} z_m(t, l)$$
$$= \alpha_{m,1} \cdot s_1(t) + \cdots + \alpha_{m,r} \cdot s_r(t) + \cdots + \alpha_{m,R} \cdot s_R(t) + v_m(t),$$
$$(1\text{-}2)$$

where

  r is the number of the electrical source; $r = 1, 2, \ldots, R$;

  $s_r(t)$ represents the enhanced stimulus-phase-locked brain activity, spontaneous brain activity, or a mixture of the spontaneous brain activities;

  $a_{m,r}$ denotes the coefficient between source #r and the point where electrode #m is placed along the scalp; and

  $v_m(t)$ represents the mixture of the sensor noise.

Obviously, the ERP data of one electrode are a mixture of many underlying sources. In Eqs. (1-1) and (1-2), the collected data and the number of electrodes are known, and the sources, number of sources, coefficients between the sources and the points where the electrodes are placed along the scalp, and the sensor noise are unknown. Furthermore, we do not know whether the different trials have different numbers of sources or whether the number of sources in the ERP data model [Eq. (1-2)] is different from that in any single trial.

1.4 Existing Problems in Conventional ERP Data Processing and Their Solutions

1.4.1 *Assumptions for the averaging step*

For the averaging step shown in Figure 1.2, the single-trial EEG data model in Eq. (1-1) in the ERP study must obey three assumptions.

(1) The artifacts are completely removed.
(2) The single-trial EEG data include randomly fluctuating spontaneous brain activity and constant brain activity, which is phase-locked to the stimulus.
(3) The sensor noise follows a Gaussian distribution.

Another fact in the single-trial EEG data modeled by Eq. (1-1) is that the phase-locked constant brain activity is much smaller than the spontaneous brain activity (Luck, 2005).

1.4.2 *Problems in the assumptions of the averaging step*

On the basis of the foregoing assumptions, averaging can enhance the common brain activity across single trials and can significantly decrease the randomly fluctuating spontaneous brain activity and sensor noise as long as the number of single trials is sufficient. The ideal conditions to achieve these assumptions are the following:

(1) The numbers of sources in any single trial are the same, which means that

$$N(1) = N(2) = \cdots = N(l) = \cdots = N(L) = R.$$

(2) The orders of the sources in any single trial are the same.

(3) $a_{m,n} \cdot s_n(t) = \frac{1}{L} \sum_{\ell=1}^{L} a_{m,n}(\ell) \cdot s_n(t, \ell)$.

Consequently, another underlying assumption is that the phase-locked constant brain activity must be larger than the mixture of the randomly fluctuating spontaneous brain activities in the ERP data modeled by Eq. (1-2) because the randomly fluctuating spontaneous brain activity does not possess similar signs, and averaging over single trials weakens it.

In practice however, many problems relative to these assumptions exist, as described below.

(1) Precisely knowing by how much the randomly fluctuating spontaneous brain activity and sensor noise have decreased is not possible.
(2) It is not possible to have the single-trial EEG be completely free of artifacts either.
(3) The number of single trials, particularly for children and patients, can be very limited.
(4) The ERP data, i.e., the averaged EEG over single trials, can still include stimulus-phase locked brain activity, mixture of spontaneous brain activities, artifacts, and sensor noise.
(5) In most cases, the stimulus-phase-locked brain activity has a smaller magnitude than the other activities in the ERP data.

Figure 1.4 shows the single-trial EEG data for 333 single trials at Fz (frontal midline of scalp) in an ERP study (Cong, Kalyakin, Li, *et al.*, 2011). Obviously, the five above-mentioned problems can all exist in the averaged EEG data over these 333 single trials.

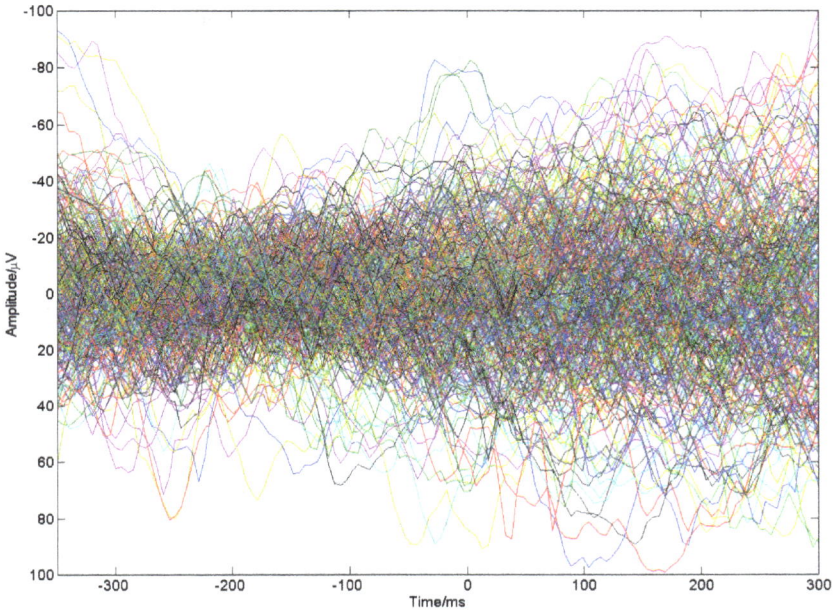

Figure 1.4 Demonstration of the single-trial EEG data of 333 single trials in the ERP study. The curves with different colors denote the different trials [adapted from Cong, Kalyakin, Li, *et al.* (2011)].

1.4.3 *Solutions*

Signal processing in an ERP study is usually applied on the continuous EEG data or concatenated single-trial EEG data (Delorme & Makeig, 2004; Luck, 2005). From the discussion in the previous section, we can conclude that further signal processing of the ERP data (i.e., averaged EEG data over single trials) is necessary to extract the ERP components.

However, the averaged EEG data over single trials are much shorter than the continuous or the concatenated single-trial EEG data. They are usually shorter than 1 s. Investigations on how to perform signal processing for such short ERP data in ERP studies are not often made, although some filtering and some time-frequency or spectral analyses have already been applied (Basar, 2004; Cohen, 2014; Freeman & Quian Quiroga, 2013).

In Chapters 2–4, we will mainly introduce the application of signal processing methods to separate the short averaged EEG data, which are a mixture of the stimulus-phase-locked brain activity, spontaneous brain activity, artifacts, and sensor noise, to extract the ERP components. The methods include the frequency-response-based wavelet filter (Cong, He, *et al.*, 2013; Cong, Huang, *et al.*, 2012; Cong, Leppänen, *et al.*, 2011), systematic ICA to extract the ERP components from the ERP data of a subject under one experimental condition (Cong, Alluri, *et al.*, 2013; Cong, He, Hämäläinen, Cichocki, & Ristaniemi, 2011; Cong, Kalyakin, Huttunen-Scott, *et al.*, 2010; Cong, Kalyakin, Li, *et al.*, 2011; Cong, Kalyakin, & Ristaniemi, 2011; Cong, Kalyakin, Zheng, & Ristaniemi, 2011; Cong, Leppänen, *et al.*, 2011), and nonnegative tensor factorization (NTF) to extract the multi-domain features of the ERPs for group-level analysis of the ERPs (Cong, Kalyakin, Phan, *et al.*, 2010; Cong, Phan, Astikainen, *et al.*, 2012; Cong, Phan, *et al.*, 2013; Cong, Phan, Lyytinen, Ristaniemi, & Cichocki, 2010; Cong, Phan, Zhao, *et al.*, 2012; Cong *et al.*, 2014). By using these approaches, the ERP data are sequentially and simultaneously filtered in the time, frequency, and space domains.

1.5 ERP Data for the Demonstration in This Book

In this study, the ERP data examples are based on auditory mismatch negativity (MMN) (Näätänen, Gaillard, & Mäntysalo, 1978; Näätänen *et al.*, 2011, 2012) and visual MMN (vMMN) (Astikainen, Cong, Ristaniemi, & Hietanen, 2013; Astikainen, Lillstrang, & Ruusuvirta, 2008). It should be noted that the research protocols for EEG data collection were approved by the local ethical committees.

MMN is an ERP with a relatively smaller amplitude. The signal processing of MMN is more critical in contrast to that of an ERP with a larger amplitude. The Appendix in this book introduces the basic knowledge on MMN, which is very important in understanding the demonstrations in Chapters 2–4.

References

Adeli, H. & Ghosh-Dastidar, S. (2010). *Automated EEG-Based Diagnosis of Neurological Disorders — Inventing the Future of Neurology*. Florida, USA: CRC Press.

Astikainen, P., Cong, F., Ristaniemi, T., & Hietanen, J. K. (2013). Event-related potentials to unattended changes in facial expressions: Detection of regularity violations or encoding of emotions? *Frontiers in Human Neuroscience, 7*, 557. Doi: 10.3389/fnhum.2013.00557; 10.3389/fnhum.2013.00557.

Astikainen, P., Lillstrang, E., & Ruusuvirta, T. (2008). Visual mismatch negativity for changes in orientation — A sensory memory-dependent response. *The European Journal of Neuroscience, 28*(11), 2319–2324. Doi: 10.1111/j.1460-9568.2008.06510.x.

Basar, E. (2004). *Memory and Brain Dynamics: Oscillations Integrating Attention, Perception, Learning, and Memory* (Vol. 1). Florida, USA: CRC Press.

Berger, H. (1929). Ueber das Elektrenkephalogramm des Menschen. *Archives fur Psychiatrie Nervenkrankheiten, 87*, 527–570.

Cohen, M. X. (2014). *Analyzing Neural Time Series Data: Theory and Practice*. Cambridge, MA: The MIT Press.

Cong, F., Alluri, V., Nandi, A. K., Toiviainen, P., Fa, R., Abu-Jamous, B., . . . Ristaniemi, T. (2013). Linking brain responses to naturalistic music through analysis of ongoing EEG and stimulus features. *IEEE Transactions on Multimedia, 15*(5), 1060–1069.

Cong, F., He, Z., Hämäläinen, J., Cichocki, A., & Ristaniemi, T. (2011). Determining the Number of Sources in High-density EEG Recordings of Event-related Potentials by Model Order Selection. *Proceedings of IEEE Workshop on Machine Learning for Signal Processing (MLSP) 2011*, Beijing, China, September 18–21, 1–6.

Cong, F., He, Z., Hämäläinen, J., Leppänen, P. H. T., Lyytinen, H., Cichocki, A., & Ristaniemi, T. (2013). Validating rationale of group-level component analysis based on estimating number of sources in EEG through model order selection. *Journal of Neuroscience Methods, 212*(1), 165–172.

Cong, F., Huang, Y., Kalyakin, I., Li, H., Huttunen-Scott, T., Lyytinen, H., & Ristaniemi, T. (2012). Frequency response based wavelet decomposition to extract children's mismatch negativity elicited by uninterrupted sound. *Journal of Medical and Biological Engineering, 32*(3), 205–214.

Cong, F., Kalyakin, I., Huttunen -Scott, T., Li, H., Lyytinen, H., & Ristaniemi, T. (2010). Single-trial based independent component analysis on mismatch negativity in children. *International Journal of Neural Systems, 20*(4), 279–292.

Cong, F., Kalyakin, I., Li, H., Huttunen-Scott, T., Huang, Y. X., Lyytinen, H., & Ristaniemi, T. (2011). Answering six questions in extracting children's mismatch negativity through combining wavelet decomposition and independent component analysis. *Cognitive Neurodynamics, 5*(4), 343–359.

Cong, F., Kalyakin, I., Phan, A. H., Cichocki, A., Huttunen-Scott, T., Lyytinen, H., & Ristaniemi, T. (2010). Extract Mismatch Negativity and P3a through Two-Dimensional Nonnegative Decomposition on Time-Frequency Represented Event-Related Potentials. In L. Zhang, J. Kwok, and B.-L. Lu (Eds.). ISNN 2010, Part II, *Lecture Notes in Computer Science, 6064*, 385–391.

Cong, F., Kalyakin, I., & Ristaniemi, T. (2011). Can back-projection fully resolve polarity indeterminacy of ICA in study of ERP? *Biomedical Signal Processing and Control, 6*(4), 422–426.

Cong, F., Kalyakin, I., Zheng, C., & Ristaniemi, T. (2011). Analysis on subtracting projection of extracted independent components from EEG recordings. *Biomedizinische Technik/Biomedical Engineering, 56*(4), 223–234.

Cong, F., Leppänen, P. H., Astikainen, P., Hämäläinen, J., Hietanen, J. K., & Ristaniemi, T. (2011). Dimension reduction: Additional benefit of an optimal filter for independent component analysis to extract event-related potentials. *Journal of Neuroscience Methods*, *201*(1), 269–280. Doi: 10.1016/j.jneumeth.2011.07.015.

Cong, F., Phan, A. H., Astikainen, P., Zhao, Q., Hietanen, J. K., Ristaniemi, T., & Cichocki, A. (2012). Multi-domain feature of event-related potential extracted by nonnegative tensor factorization: 5 vs. 14 electrodes EEG data. In A. Cichocki *et al.* (Eds.). LVA/ICA 2012, *Lecture Notes in Computer Science*, *7191*, 502–510.

Cong, F., Phan, A. H., Astikainen, P., Zhao, Q., Wu, Q., Hietanen, J. K., . . . Cichocki, A. (2013). Multi-domain feature extraction for small event-related potentials through nonnegative multi-way array decomposition from low dense array EEG. *International Journal of Neural Systems*, *23*(2(1350006)), 1–18. Doi: 10.1142/S0129065713500068.

Cong, F., Phan, A. H., Lyytinen, H., Ristaniemi, T., & Cichocki, A. (2010). Classifying Healthy Children and Children with Attention Deficit through Features Derived from Sparse and Nonnegative Tensor Factorization Using Event-related Potential. In V. Vigneron *et al.* (Eds.). LVA/ICA 2010, *Lecture Notes in Computer Science*, *6365*, 620–628.

Cong, F., Phan, A. H., Zhao, Q., Huttunen-Scott, T., Kaartinen, J., Ristaniemi, T., . . . Cichocki, A. (2012). Benefits of multi-domain feature of mismatch negativity extracted by non-negative tensor factorization from EEG collected by low-density array. *International Journal of Neural Systems*, *22*(6-1250025), 1–19. Doi: 10.1142/S0129065712500256.

Cong, F., Zhou, G., Astikainen, P., Zhao, Q., Wu, Q., Nandi, A. K., . . . Cichocki, A. (2014). Low-rank approximation based nonnegative multi-way array decomposition on event-related potentials. *International Journal of Neural Systems*. Doi: 10.1142/S012906571440005X.

Davis, H., Davis, P. A., Loomis, A. L., Harvey, E. N., & Hobart, G. (1939). Electrical reactions of the human brain to auditory stimulation during sleep. *Journal of Neurophysiology*, 2, 500–514.

Delorme, A. & Makeig, S. (2004). EEGLAB: An open source toolbox for analysis of single-trial EEG dynamics including independent component analysis. *Journal of Neuroscience Methods*, *134*(1), 9–21. Doi: 10.1016/j.jneumeth.2003.10.009.

Dmochowski, J. P., Sajda, P., Dias, J., & Parra, L. C. (2012). Correlated components of ongoing EEG point to emotionally laden attention — A possible marker of engagement? *Frontiers in Human Neuroscience*, *6*, 112. Doi: 10.3389/fnhum.2012.00112; 10.3389/fnhum.2012.00112.

Freeman, W. J. & Quian Quiroga, R. (2013). *Imaging Brain Function With EEG: Advanced Temporal and Spatial Analysis of Electroencephalographic Signals*. New York: Springer.

Jung, T. P., Makeig, S., Westerfield, M., Townsend, J., Courchesne, E., & Sejnowski, T. J. (2000). Removal of eye activity artifacts from visual event-related potentials in normal and clinical subjects. *Clinical Neurophysiology: Official Journal of the International Federation of Clinical Neurophysiology*, *111*(10), 1745–1758.

Luck, S. J. (2005). *An Introduction to the Event-Related Potential Technique* Cambridge, MA: The MIT Press.

Makeig, S., Jung, T. P., Bell, A. J., Ghahremani, D., & Sejnowski, T. J. (1997). Blind separation of auditory event-related brain responses into independent components. *Proceedings of the National Academy of Sciences of the United States of America*, *94*(20), 10979–10984.

Morup, M., Hansen, L. K., & Arnfred, S. M. (2007). ERPWAVELAB a toolbox for multichannel analysis of time-frequency transformed event related potentials. *Journal of Neuroscience Methods*, *161*(2), 361–368. Doi: 10.1016/j.jneumeth.2006.11.008.

Näätänen, R., Gaillard, A. W., & Mäntysalo, S. (1978). Early selective-attention effect on evoked potential reinterpreted. *Acta Psychologica*, *42*(4), 313–329.

Näätänen, R., Kujala, T., Escera, C., Baldeweg, T., Kreegipuu, K., Carlson, C., & Ponton, C. (2012). The mismatch negativity (MMN) — A unique window to disturbed central auditory processing in ageing and different clinical conditions. *Clinical Neurophysiology: Official Journal of the International Federation of Clinical Neurophysiology*, *123*, 424–458.

Näätänen, R., Kujala, T., Kreegipuu, K., Carlson, S., Escera, C., Baldeweg, T., & Ponton, C. (2011). The mismatch negativity: an index of cognitive decline in neuropsychiatric and neurological diseases and in ageing. *Brain: A Journal of Neurology*, 134(Pt 12), 3432–3450. Doi: 10.1093/brain/awr064.

Niedermeyer, E. & Lopes da Silva, F. (2004). *Electroencephalography: Basic Principles, Clinical Applications, and Related Fields*. Baltimore, MD: Williams & Wilkins.

Nunez, P. & Srinivasan, R. (2005). *Electric Fields of the Brain: The Neurophysics of EEG* (Vol. 2). New York: Oxford University Press.

Onton, J., Westerfield, M., Townsend, J., & Makeig, S. (2006). Imaging human EEG dynamics using independent component analysis. *Neuroscience and Biobehavioral Reviews*, *30*(6), 808–822. Doi: 10.1016/j.neubiorev.2006.06.007.

Quian Quiroga, R. & Garcia, H. (2003). Single-trial event-related potentials with wavelet denoising. *Clinical Neurophysiology: Official Journal Of The International Federation of Clinical Neurophysiology*, *114*(2), 376–390.

Sanei, S. & Chambers, J. A. (2007). *EEG Signal Processing*. Wiley.

Talsma, D. (2008). Auto-adaptive averaging: Detecting artifacts in event-related potential data using a fully automated procedure. *Psychophysiology*, *45*(2), 216–228. Doi: 10.1111/j.1469-8986.2007.00612.x.

Tan, D. S. & Nijholt, A. (2010). *Brain–Computer Interfaces: Applying our Minds to Human–Computer Interaction*. London: Springer.

Chapter 2

Wavelet Filter Design Based on Frequency Responses for Filtering ERP Data With Duration of One Epoch

In this chapter, we introduce the definition of correlation, impulse response, and frequency response of a digital filter; the moving-average model-based finite impulse response (FIR) digital filter; the discrete Fourier transform (DFT)-based digital filter; and the wavelet transform-based wavelet filter. In addition, we introduce the methods for interpreting all the filters by correlation and designing the wavelet filter in terms of the frequency response of a digital filter.

2.1 Correlation

Correlation is a common term and an academic and technical one. In contrast to many other technical terms, e.g., filter, convolution, transform, and so on, we believe that understanding correlation is much easier. Therefore, we will illustrate the different filters in terms of correlation.

Given two time series $\alpha(t)$ and $\beta(t)$, the cross-correlation sequence (Mitra, 2005) is defined as

$$r_{\alpha\beta}(\tau) = \sum_{t=-\infty}^{\infty} \alpha(t) \cdot \beta(t-\tau), \quad \tau = 0, \pm 1, 2, \ldots \qquad (2\text{-}1)$$

where $\alpha(t)$ is called the reference signal. In particular, when $\tau = 0$, we define the correlation between the two time series $\alpha(t)$ and $\beta(t)$ as follows:

$$r_{\alpha\beta} = \sum_{t=-\infty}^{\infty} \alpha(t) \cdot \beta(t). \tag{2-2}$$

Indeed, the correlation of the two time series is simply their inner product. When the mean and variance of each time series are respectively 0 and 1, the correlation is simply the correlation coefficient.

2.2 Impulse Response and Frequency Response

The impulse response of a digital filter is the output of the filter when the input is a unit impulse (Mitra, 2005). Figure 2.1 shows the unit impulse and the impulse response of a digital filter. They are generated by the FDALTOOL function of MATLAB (The Mathworks, Inc., Natick, MA, 2010).

The impulse response is very important for a digital filter, and it can assist in determining the digital filter properties. The Fourier transform (introduced later in this chapter) of the impulse response generates the

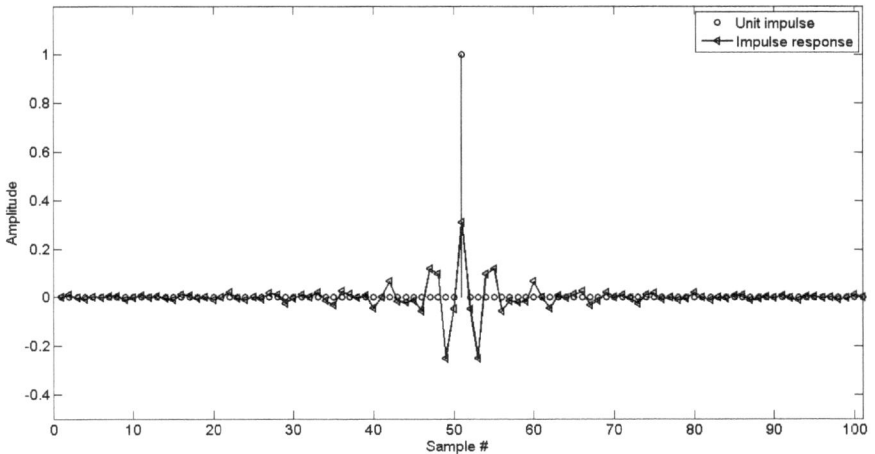

Figure 2.1   Demonstration of the unit impulse and impulse response of a band-pass FIR digital filter. The number of orders is 100, the sampling frequency is 200 Hz, the pass band is from 40 to 70 Hz, and the stop bands are at 39 and 71 Hz. The least square method is applied in designing the filter.

(a)

(b)

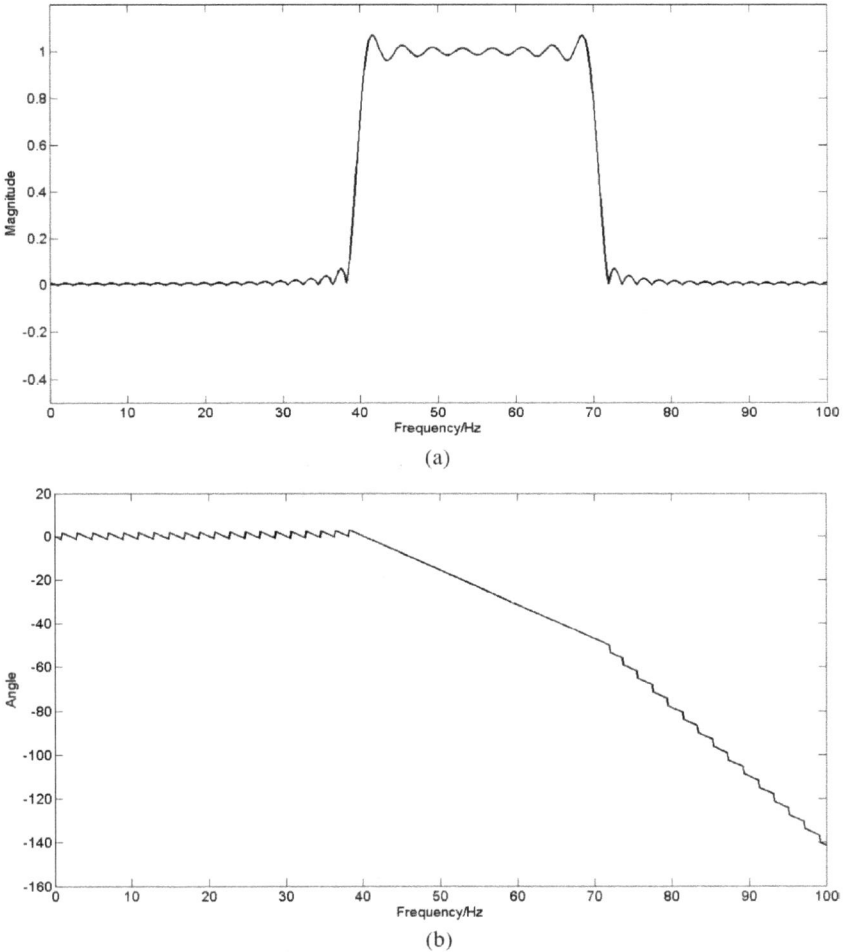

Figure 2.2 Frequency response of the digital filter shown in Figure 2.1. (a) Magnitude response. (b) Phase response.

Note: The filter is not well designed.

frequency response, which includes the magnitude and phase responses (Mitra, 2005). The magnitude and phase responses are respectively the absolute and phase values of the Fourier transform of the impulse response. Figure 2.2 shows the frequency response of the digital filter presented in Figure 2.1.

2.3 Moving-Average Model-Based FIR Digital Filter

2.3.1 *Interpreting the digital filter in terms of correlation*

The moving-average model is an expression of the FIR filter (Mitra, 2005).
It is expressed as

$$y(t) = \sum_{\tau=0}^{P} h(\tau) \cdot x(t - \tau), \qquad (2\text{-}3)$$

where $\tau = 0, 1, 2, \ldots, P$; $x(t)$ is the input to the filter; $h(\tau)$ is the filter
impulse response with length P [an example of $h(\tau)$ is shown in Figure 2.1];
$y(t)$ is the filter output; and P is the order of the filter. Usually, the digital
filter is illustrated as a convolution between the impulse response and the
input signal. Indeed, it can be interpreted using the correlation. If we define
$\alpha(\tau) = h(\tau)$ and $\beta_t(\tau) = x(t - \tau)$, Eq. (2-3) can be transformed into

$$y(t) = r_{\alpha\beta_t} = \sum_{\tau=0}^{P} \alpha(\tau) \cdot \beta_t(\tau). \qquad (2\text{-}4)$$

Then, the filter output is certainly the correlation between the impulse
response $\alpha(\tau)$ and sample sequence $\beta_t(\tau)$ at each sample index t. The sample sequence $\beta_t(\tau)$ includes the current input and the past P inputs to the
filter. When the magnitude of the correlation at one sample index t is high,
the sample sequence is similar to the impulse response at this sample index t.
Therefore, the impulse response property and the filter order (i.e., times of
delay) determine the FIR digital filter characteristics.

2.3.2 *Problems of the digital filter in removing artifacts*
and their solutions

Both FIR and infinite impulse response (IIR) digital filters have been
extensively used to remove artifacts and noise in electroencephalography
(EEG) data. The IIR filter is based on the autoregressive and moving-average
model (Mitra, 2005) and can be interpreted using the correlation. Both filters
are usually employed in event-related potential (ERP) studies on continuous
or concatenated single-trial EEG data, as shown in Figure 1.2 (Luck, 2005).
By taking the FIR filter as an example, we briefly introduce the problem of
the FIR filter application in ERP studies.

From the signal processing viewpoint, the pass band of the magnitude response is usually expected to be as flat as possible, the transitional band is attenuated as fast as possible, and the pass band of the phase response is as linear as possible (Mitra, 2005). However, in practice, "keeping offline filtering to a minimum" is recommended by Luck (2005) when a digital filter is applied to filter the above-mentioned EEG data. This is because a digital filter that causes sharp attenuation of the magnitude response in the transitional band could practically distort the ERP waveforms (Luck, 2005). Such contradiction has never been sufficiently discussed from the viewpoint of signal processing. Interestingly, understanding such problem is straightforward using correlation.

Equation (2-4) shows that the impulse response of a filter does not change when the sample index t input changes. For the correlation operation, we expect that the two time series to be correlated with each other are stationary; otherwise, the correlation result would not be precise. In Eq. (2-4), the two time series are the impulse response and the sample sequence. For a given digital filter, the impulse response is already fixed and usually stationary, as shown in Figure 2.1. In the continuous or concatenated single-trial EEG data, artifacts tend to appear. For each EEG data sample, a sample sequence $\beta_t(\tau)$ exists according to Eq. (2-4). As mentioned earlier, the sample sequence consists of the current input $x(t)$ of the filter and the previous input $x(t - \tau)$, $\tau = 1, 2, \ldots, P$. Obviously, the sample sequence can be either stationary or nonstationary, as shown in Figure 1.2. When many artifacts appear, the correlation between the impulse response and sample sequence $\beta_t(\tau)$ will not be precise, resulting in technical artifacts; thus, the application of the digital filter to the continuous or concatenated single-trial EEG data should be minimal.

If the digital filter is applied to the EEG data of one single trial instead of the continuous or concatenated single-trial EEG data, the problem can be alleviated to some extent. In ERP experiments, the duration of one single trial is very short (usually less than 1 s). With a sampling frequency of 500 Hz, the number of samples can be a few hundreds only. For the FIR and IIR filters, the main approach is to increase the order of the filter (i.e., increasing) to achieve a flat pass band and sharp attenuation of the transitional band of the magnitude response. However, in some filter design methods, the filter order of a zero-phase FIR filter is limited to be smaller than one-third of the number of samples in the signal in MATLAB (The Mathworks, Inc., Natick, MA, 2010). Figure 2.2 shows that the filter is designed at order $P = 101$. The filter is not satisfactory because of the ripple in the pass band of the magnitude response. This deficiency motivates us to study the filtering of EEG data with a duration of one epoch in ERP experiments.

2.4 DFT-Based Digital Filter

2.4.1 *Definition of DFT*

Given length-T discrete sequence $x(t)$, $t = 0, 1, 2, \ldots, T-1$, the K-point ($K \geq T$) DFT is defined as follows:

$$X(k) = \sum_{t=0}^{T-1} x(t) \cdot e^{-j2\pi \frac{k}{K}t}, \tag{2-5}$$

where $k = 0, 1, 2, \ldots, K-1$, $j^2 = -1$, and e is the Euler's number (2.718......).

2.4.2 *Interpreting DFT using correlation*

Equation (2-5) can be written as

$$X(k) = r_{\alpha\beta_k} - j \cdot r_{\alpha\theta_k} = \sum_{t=0}^{T-1} \alpha(t) \cdot \beta_k(t) - j \cdot \sum_{t=0}^{T-1} \alpha(t) \cdot \theta_k(t), \tag{2-6}$$

$$e^{-j2\pi \frac{k}{K}t} = \cos\left(2\pi \frac{k}{K}t\right) - j \cdot \sin\left(2\pi \frac{k}{K}t\right) = \beta_k(t) - j \cdot \theta_k(t), \tag{2-7}$$

where $\alpha(t) = x(t)$, $\beta_k(t) = \cos(2\pi \frac{k}{K}t)$, and $\theta_k(t) = \sin(2\pi \frac{k}{K}t)$. Obviously, the signal to be transformed by the correlation operation is the reference signal. $\beta_k(t)$ and $\theta_k(t)$ are the cosine and sine functions at a given frequency bin. Therefore, the Fourier transform is simply the correlation between the signal and the cosine and sine functions at a given frequency. A high correlation at a given frequency indicates that the signal carries information on that frequency. Figure 2.3 shows an example of the spontaneous EEG at the alpha band (Berger, 1929).

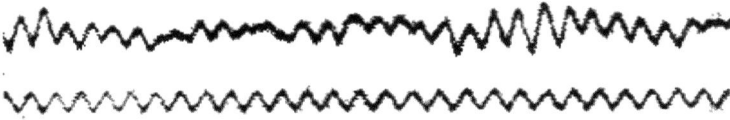

Figure 2.3 Spontaneous EEG at the alpha band and the 10-Hz cosine function (Berger, 1929).

2.4.3 *DFT-based digital filter*

Equation (2-5) shows that after the time-domain signal $x(t)$ is transformed by DFT, a complex-valued sequence $X(k)$ is produced in the frequency domain with $k = 0, 1, 2, \ldots, K-1$. The sampling frequency Fs is uniformly divided into K parts. Therefore, we can identify which frequency bin corresponds to which frequency. Using a band-pass filter, we want to remove some frequency components from the input signal. This can be achieved by the following approach:

(1) Apply the DFT on the signal.
(2) Set $X(k)$, which is outside the pass band, as zero to create a new frequency-domain sequence $Y(k)$. Hence, the $X(k)$ and $Y(k)$ characteristics would be that they are identical within the pass band and different outside the pass band.
(3) Apply inverse DFT on $Y(k)$ to obtain the filtered signal $y(t)$. Therefore, the theoretical difference between $x(t)$ and $y(t)$ is that $y(t)$ only carries the frequency components of $x(t)$ in the pass band of the filter.

Figure 2.4 shows the frequency response of the DFT-based digital filter. In contrast to the frequency response of the FIR digital filter shown in Figure 2.2, the magnitude response of the DFT-based digital filter attenuates much faster in the transitional band. In addition, the phase response of the DFT-based digital filter is more linear, which is clearly the advantage of the DFT-based digital filter over the FIR digital filter when both filters are used to filter EEG data with a duration of one single trial in ERP experiments.

The order of the FIR digital filter tends to be limited by the short duration of the EEG data in this case. Therefore, the duration of the impulse response of the FIR digital filter is also limited. However, the duration of the impulse response of the DFT-based digital filter is not strictly limited by the length of

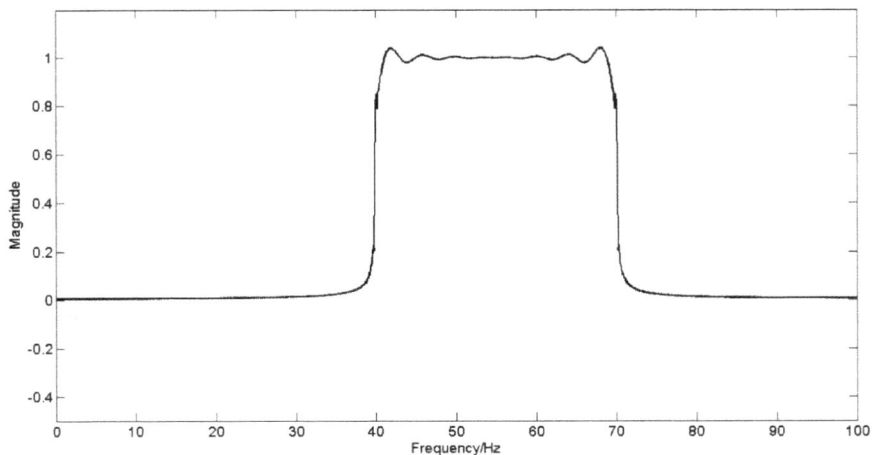

(a)

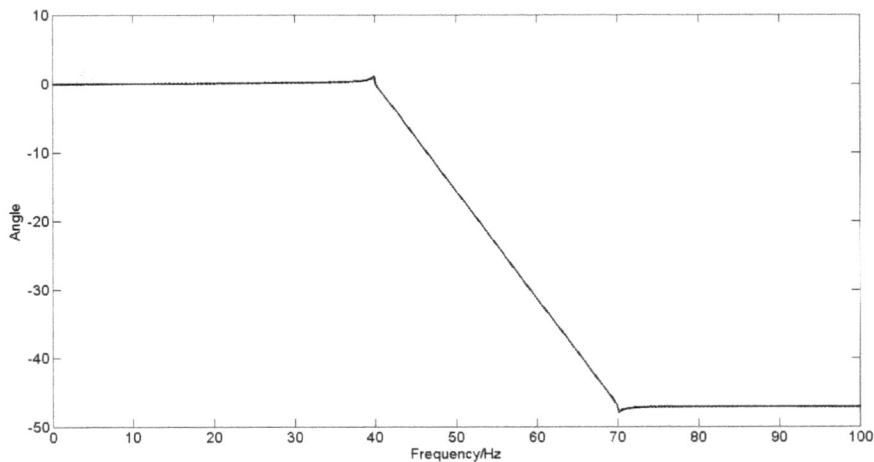

(b)

Figure 2.4   Frequency response of the DFT-based digital filter. (a) Magnitude response. (b) Phase response. The sampling frequency of the signal is 200 Hz, and the pass band is from 40 to 70 Hz.

the input signal. In actual case, such difference results in different filtering performance. Hereinafter, we use "DFT filter" to denote the DFT-based digital filter for simplicity.

2.4.4 *Problems of the DFT filter and their corresponding solutions*

As mentioned earlier, Fourier transform is the correlation between the signal and the cosine and the sine functions at a given frequency. The cosine and sine functions are stationary time series. However, the EEG data of a single trial in ERP experiments do not always mean to be stationary. Therefore, when the EEG data of a single trial are nonstationary, the DFT-based Fourier is not precise. Furthermore, Eq. (2-7) shows that the Fourier transform is indeed based on the cosine and sine function models. If the model can be changed to adapt more to nonstationary signals, the transform will become more accurate.

Moreover, from the DFT definition in Eq. (2-5), we can state that the K frequency bins are uniformly distributed over the frequency range from 0 Hz to the sampling frequency. This means that the frequency resolution in the DFT is constant regardless of whether the frequency is high or low. In reality, a high-frequency resolution is expected for the low-frequency components. Similarly, a low-frequency resolution is expected for the high-frequency components. For example, in the theta band that ranges from 4 to 8 Hz, we expect to know the frequency components at 4, 4.5, and 5 Hz, etc. Beyond 40 Hz, knowing the frequency components at 40, 42, and 44 Hz, etc. would be satisfactory. This condition motivates the study of variable-frequency resolution when the time-domain signal is transformed into the frequency domain.

Furthermore, in ERP studies, the band-pass digital filter extracts the frequency components from a certain frequency band and uses them to reconstruct the desired ERP signal. This method is extensively used owing to its robustness, simplicity, and low computation cost. However, the overlapping frequency components of the source signals within the pass band of a digital filter cannot be separated. Therefore, the output of a digital filter is a mixture of various source signals.

Next, we will show that the wavelet transform (Daubechies, 1992) is a practical choice in resolving the digital filter problems.

2.5 Wavelet Transform

2.5.1 *Definition of wavelet transform*

The wavelet transform includes the continuous waveform transform (CWT) and discrete wavelet transform (DWT) (Daubechies, 1992; Mallat, 1999). The definition of CWT with length-T discrete sequence $x(t)(t = 0, 1, \ldots, T - 1)$ is expressed as follows:

$$\text{CWT}(a, b) = \frac{1}{\sqrt{|a|}} \sum_{t=0}^{T-1} x(t)\psi\left(\frac{t - b}{a}\right), \qquad (2\text{-}8)$$

where $x(t)$ is the signal to be transformed and a and b are the so-called scaling (reciprocal of the frequency) and time location or shifting parameters, respectively. Therefore, $\psi(t)$ is the mother wavelet, and $\psi(\frac{t-b}{a})$ is the shifted and scaled wavelet. Figure 2.5 shows one example.

Because a and b can be defined using any possible rational numbers, calculating the wavelet coefficients becomes very computationally expensive. Instead, if the scales and shifts based on the power of two (so-called dyadic scales and positions) are selected, then the wavelet analysis will be much more efficient. Mallat first proposed this idea (Mallat, 1989). The DWT of

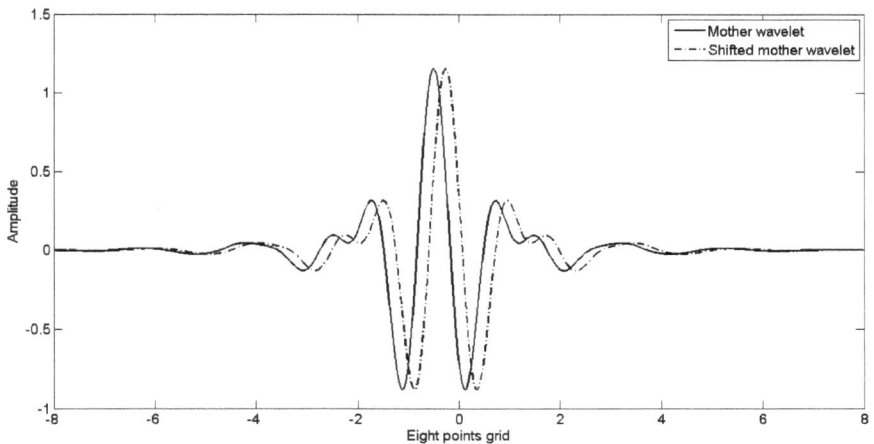

Figure 2.5   Mother wavelet and shifted mother wavelet. The above example is a Meyer wavelet.

length-T discrete sequence $x(t)$ $(t = 0, 1, 2, \ldots, T-1)$ is expressed as

$$\text{DWT}(n, m) = \frac{1}{\sqrt{|2^n|}} \sum_{t=0}^{T-1} x(t) \psi \left(\frac{t - 2^n \cdot m}{2^n} \right), \tag{2-9}$$

where a and b in the CWT are replaced by 2^n and $2^n \cdot m$, respectively; n and m are integers.

We should note that the difference in the CWT and DWT is not in the signal (whether continuous or discrete) to be transformed but in the scale and shift parameters. In the CWT, the parameters are continuous, whereas they are discrete in the DWT.

2.5.2 Interpreting the wavelet transform using correlation

Equation (2-8) can be written as

$$\text{CWT}(a, b) = \frac{1}{\sqrt{|a|}} r_{\alpha \beta_{a,b}} = \frac{1}{\sqrt{|a|}} \sum_{t=0}^{T-1} \alpha(t) \cdot \beta_{a,b}(t), \tag{2-10}$$

where $\alpha(t) = x(t)$, and $\beta_{a,b}(t) = \psi(\frac{t-b}{a})$. Therefore, given scale a and shift b, the wavelet transform is the scaled correlation between signal $x(t)$ and the wavelets, which are the scaled and shifted mother wavelets. The signal to be transformed is also the reference signal.

2.5.3 Differences between the Fourier and wavelet transforms

In accordance with Eqs. (2-6) and (2-10), the correlation operation in the Fourier transform is performed at every frequency bin; that in the wavelet transform is performed at every possible scale and shift point. Therefore, the time mode disappears after the Fourier transform, and only the frequency mode is generated; however, the time mode remains after the wavelet transform, and the frequency mode is generated. Thus, the Fourier transform is used only for spectrum analysis, and the wavelet transform is used for time-frequency analysis.

From the definition of the K-point DFT, the frequency bin index k should be an integer and uniformly distributed from 0 to $K-1$. In the CWT, a can be any rational number, whereas in the DWT, a is usually associated with the power of two. Therefore, the frequency resolution in the Fourier transform is fixed but that in the wavelet transform can be variable. Using the wavelet transform, we can obtain a higher frequency resolution in the low-frequency band and a lower frequency resolution in the high-frequency band.

Figures 2.3 and 2.5 show that the Fourier basis (i.e., sine or cosine function) at any given frequency bin does not change over time, but the wavelet basis changes because of *b* in the CWT and DWT. Therefore, the correlation between the reference signal (i.e., the signal to be transformed) and the wavelet transform basis (i.e., the scaled and shifted mother wavelet) can be more accurate in contrast to that in the Fourier transform provided that the wavelet is appropriately selected.

2.5.4 *Implementation of DWT*

Mallat developed a very efficient method of implementing this scheme by passing the signal through a series of low-pass (LP) and high-pass (HP) filter pairs (Mallat, 1989). The pairs are usually called quadrature mirror filters. This procedure is shown in Figure 2.6 (Ocak, 2009).

In the first step of the DWT, the signal is simultaneously passed through the LP and HP filters with a cutoff frequency of one-half of the sampling frequency *Fs*. The outputs of the LP and HP filters are called the approximation and detail coefficients, respectively. Meanwhile, a downsampling procedure with a factor of two is also applied. Therefore, for the approximation coefficients in the first level, the sampling frequency is approximately *Fs*/2. In the DWT, only the approximation coefficients are further decomposed. Hence, in the second step, the approximation coefficients in the first level are decomposed into the approximation and detail coefficients in the second level. The sampling frequency of the

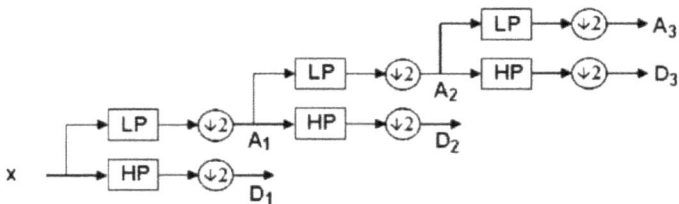

Figure 2.6   Example of the DWT implementation [adapted from Ocak (2009)].

approximation coefficients in the second level becomes approximately $Fs/4$. The same procedure is repeated for the second-level approximation coefficients in the third-level decomposition. Therefore, if the signal is decomposed into more levels, the sampling frequency of the approximation coefficients will increasingly become smaller.

We should note that in the wavelet packet decomposition, both approximation and detail coefficients are decomposed (Mallat, 1999). The illustration for the DWT in Figure 2.6 is very fundamental. In the 1990s, the development of wavelet transform was dramatic. Many derivatives for the implementation of DWT existed (Mallat, 1999). For conciseness and simplicity, we did not consider them in this book.

2.6 Wavelet Filter Design Based on Frequency Response

The Fourier and wavelet transforms have been extensively used in the spectral and time-frequency analyses of ERP data with a duration of one epoch and short spontaneous EEG data (Cohen, 2014; Freeman & Quian Quiroga, 2013). Therefore, they can also be applied to filter short ERP/EEG data. As mentioned earlier, these methods are superior over the moving-average-model-based FIR filters. The DFT filter was introduced in Section 2.4. In the next section, we introduce the design of an appropriate wavelet filter.

2.6.1 *Introduction to wavelet filter*

The wavelet filter exploits both the temporal and frequency properties of a signal. It has been used in analyzing biomedical signals with various wavelets (Adeli, Zhou, & Dadmehr, 2003; Atienza, Cantero, & Quian Quiroga, 2005; Bostanov & Kotchoubey 2006; Burger *et al.*, 2007; Cong *et al.*, 2012; Jongsma *et al.*, 2006; Quian Quiroga & Garcia, 2003; Wilson, 2004).

The wavelet filter is usually expressed in terms of the DWT. Therefore, the DWT implementation is the basis for the design of the wavelet filter. The four steps in the wavelet filter design are briefly described as follows:

(1) Determination of the number of levels L for the wavelet decomposition, as shown in Figure 2.6.

(2) Implementation of the wavelet decomposition using a chosen wavelet and the number of levels.
(3) Selection of the detail coefficients at some levels.
(4) Reconstruction of the desired signal to complete the wavelet filter.

2.6.2 *Key issues in the wavelet filter design*

In contrast to the design of a Fourier transform-based digital filter, that of the wavelet filter can be much more complicated and can be very sensitive to many parameters. Three key issues exist for the wavelet decomposition.

(1) How many levels should be used?
(2) Which levels of detail coefficients should be selected?
(3) Which wavelet should be chosen?

Next, we analyze the current solutions for each key issue, point out the existing problems, and present new solutions.

2.6.3 *Determination of the number of levels*

2.6.3.1 *Existing problem and current solution*

The first issue in Section 2.6.2 is clearly related to the number of samples in a signal. The number of levels should be not more than $\log_2 N$ (where N is the number of samples). This criterion has been widely used in biomedical signal processing since the 1990s (Tikkanen & Sellin, 1997). The main problem here is that the spectral property of the signal is not considered at all when the number of levels is selected using this method.

2.6.3.2 *New solution*

In practice, the spectral property of the signal to be analyzed should be better considered before determining the number of levels of the wavelet decomposition. For example, the ERP spectrum is in the very low-frequency band, and key energy of the ERP usually falls below the 15-Hz frequency. Therefore, in the final level of wavelet decomposition, we expect to have the sampling frequency divided into frequency bins with a resolution of 1 Hz or even higher. Hence, by considering the one-epoch duration (1 s) in ERP experiments, we suggest the use of the following criterion to determine the number of levels of the wavelet decomposition:

$$L \approx \log_2 Fs. \tag{2-11}$$

2.6.4 *Frequency division at different DWT levels: Overlapped frequency contents at different levels*

We have learned a critical misunderstanding of the LP and HP filters in the wavelet decomposition. The frequency contents of the approximation and detail coefficients at one level are usually assumed to not overlap in the frequency domain, and those of the detail coefficients at different levels are assumed to also not overlap in the frequency domain (Ocak, 2009). This assumption indicates that the pass bands of the LP and HP filters do not overlap. In accordance with this concept, the frequency contents of the approximation and the detail coefficients are believed to range respectively from 0 to $Fs/8$ Hz and from $Fs/8$ to $Fs/4$ Hz (Ocak, 2009), as shown in Figure 2.6. In the following, we show that such frequency division is not precise.

The wavelet filter can be regarded as a special digital filter. To obtain its digital-filter property, the frequency response of the filter should be calculated. Therefore, when the detail coefficients at one level are used for signal reconstruction, the magnitude response of the filter frequency response allows examination of the frequency contents of the detail coefficients at that level.

Figure 2.7 shows the magnitude responses of the wavelet filter frequency responses of wavelet filters when the detail coefficients at each of some levels are used for the signal reconstruction. Obviously, the frequency contents of the detail coefficients of some levels largely overlap with each other and the degrees of overlapping of the different wavelets can be different as well. This result indicates that the previous frequency division approach by the DWT is not precise.

Indeed, wavelet decomposition based on the DWT is similar to a digital filter bank that includes many LP and HP digital filters. In digital filters, the pass bands of the LP and HP digital filters theoretically do not overlap. The pass bands of the LP and HP filters in the wavelet decomposition can overlap with each other owing to the wavelet properties.

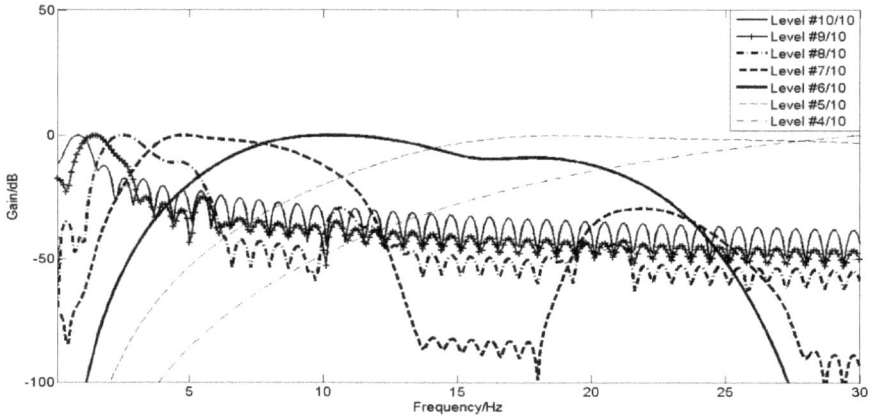

(a)

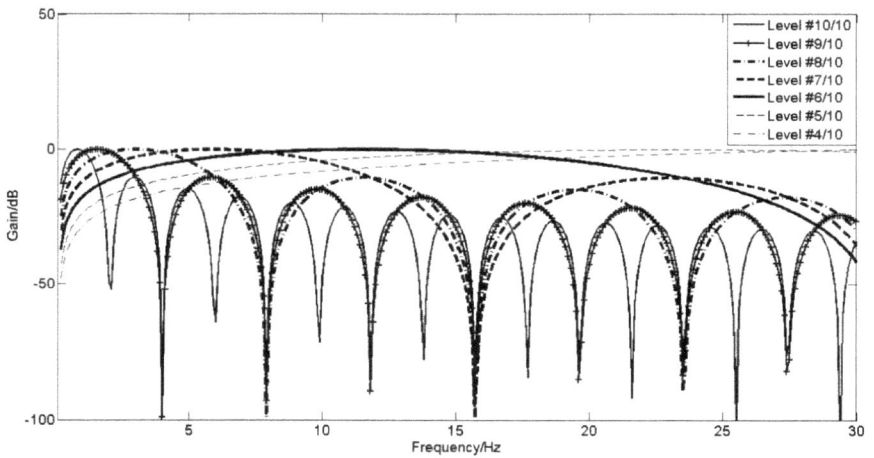

(b)

Figure 2.7 Examples of magnitude response of wavelet filters (the detail coefficients of each level are used for signal reconstruction). (a) Wavelet rbio6.8. (b) Wavelet rbio1.1. The duration of the unit impulse is 1400 ms (−700 to 700 ms). The sampling frequency of the unit impulse is 1000 Hz, and the number of levels for the decomposition is 10 according to Eq. (2-11). The level number indicated in the figure means that the detail coefficients at that level are used for signal reconstruction. Because the frequency contents of an ERP are usually smaller than 30 Hz, we only show the magnitude responses below 30 Hz.

2.6.5 *Frequency division in the first level of DWT: The cutoff frequency of the LP and HP filters is Fs/2 instead of Fs/4*

In particular, the frequency division at the first level in previous DWT studies was wrong. For example, the frequency contents of the approximation coefficients were assumed to be from 0 to $Fs/4$ Hz, and those of the detail coefficients were from $Fs/4$ to $Fs/2$ Hz (Ocak, 2009). This means that the cutoff frequency of the LP and HP filters is $Fs/4$ Hz (Ocak, 2009).

Such frequency division at the first level of the DWT is wrong. The sampling frequency of the signal is Fs, and the signal is usually LP-filtered with a cutoff frequency much smaller than $Fs/2$ according to the sampling theorem (Mitra, 2005). Therefore, the frequency contents of the approximation and detail coefficients should be approximately from 0 to $Fs/2$ Hz and from $Fs/2$ to Fs Hz at the first level, respectively. The latter is already removed when the signal is preprocessed.

Figure 2.8 shows the frequency contents of the detail coefficients at each of the first several levels in the DWT. The contents are determined by the frequency responses of the wavelet filter. Because of the Fourier transform property, we cannot obtain the frequency contents beyond half of the sampling frequency, and the frequency contents are symmetric with respect to the center at half of the sampling frequency (Mitra, 2005). The frequency contents of the detail coefficients at level #2 are clearly below $Fs/2$ Hz but not below $Fs/4$ Hz [$Fs/4$ Hz was reported previously (Ocak, 2009)]. Therefore, we cannot expect that the frequency contents of the detail coefficients at level #1 are all below $Fs/2$ Hz.

2.6.6 *Selection of the detail coefficients at some levels for signal reconstruction*

2.6.6.1 *Existing problem and current solution*

For the second issue in Section 2.6.2, the most commonly used methods are the calculation of the correlation coefficient of the selected wavelet coefficients and the assumed desired signal (Burger *et al.*, 2007), and the frequency band computation at each level according to the frequency division from the association of the sampling frequency and the number of levels of decomposition (Ocak, 2009; Wang, Miao, & Kang, 2009).

(a)

(b)

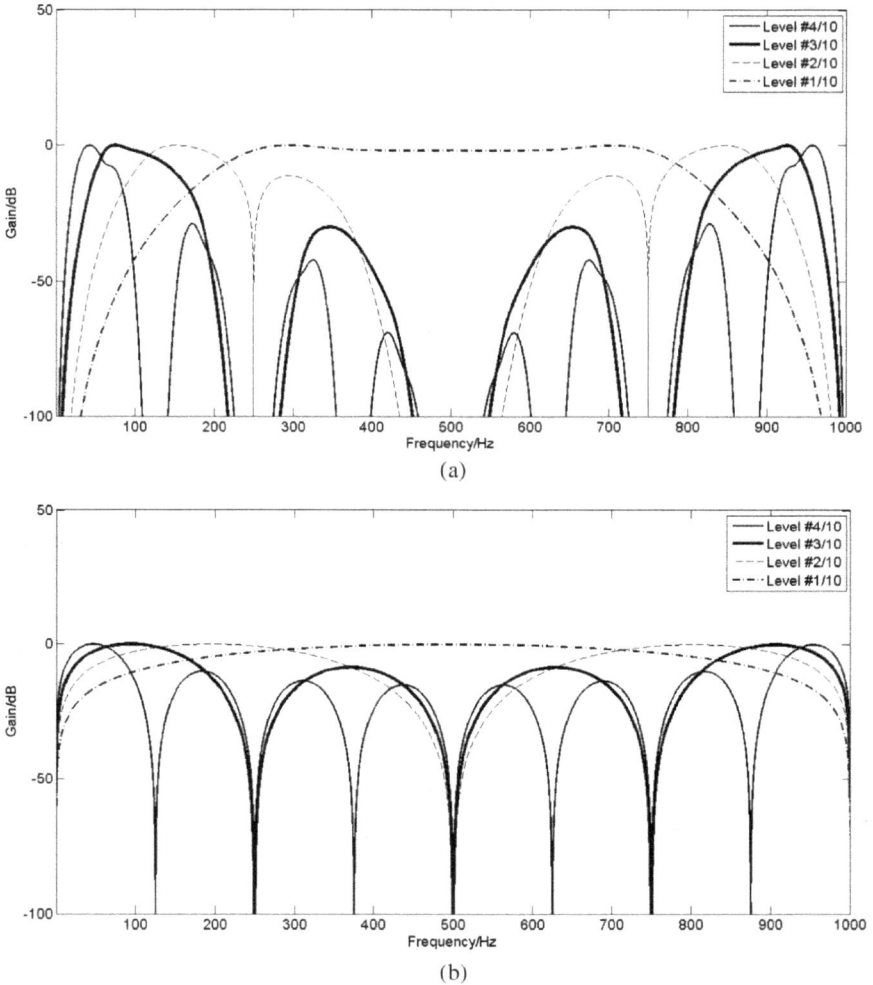

Figure 2.8 Examples of the magnitude responses of the wavelet filters (the detail coefficients at each of the first levels are used for the signal reconstruction). (a) wavelet rbio6.8. (b) Wavelet rbio1.1. The duration of the unit impulse is 1400 ms (−700 to 700 ms). The sampling frequency of the unit impulse is 1000 Hz, and the number of levels for the decomposition is 10 according to Eq. (2-11). The level number listed in the figure indicates that the detail coefficients at that level are used for the signal reconstruction.

For the first method, the coefficients, which are more correlated with the desired signal, are selected. If the desired signal is known, the first method can be very effective. However, the desired signal is rarely known in practice. Therefore, this method is not realistic in most cases. The second method does not consider the information on the wavelet at all, which means that such method is not optimal.

2.6.6.2 *New solution*

On the basis of the results shown in Figure 2.7, the frequency contents in the detail coefficients should be defined by the frequency response of the wavelet filter in which the detail coefficients at each level are used for signal reconstruction. Therefore, selection of the detail coefficients at the level should be performed according to the frequency response properties of the wavelet filter and the spectral property of the desired signal.

2.6.7 *Choosing the wavelet for the wavelet filter in ERP studies*

2.6.7.1 *Existing problem and current solution*

For the third issue in Section 2.6.2, some information-theory-based methods have been proposed (Coifman & Wickerhauser, 1992; Donoho & Johnstone, 1994). However, they are not widely used in biomedical signal processing when the wavelet transform is applied. This issue is usually dealt with by the empirical experience of the users, which is often subjective.

2.6.7.2 *New solution*

This book is about ERP data processing. Therefore, we recommend the investigation of the impulse response and the frequency response of a wavelet filter to choose the appropriate wavelet, which takes into account the ERP spectral property. Figures 2.9 and 2.10 show examples in choosing the suitable wavelet in terms of this criterion.

Figure 2.9 shows the unit impulse and impulse responses of three wavelet filters using three different wavelets, aimed at filtering the ERP data. Consequently, we can immediately reject the reverse biorthogonal wavelet "rbio1.1" because the impulse response indicates that the wavelet

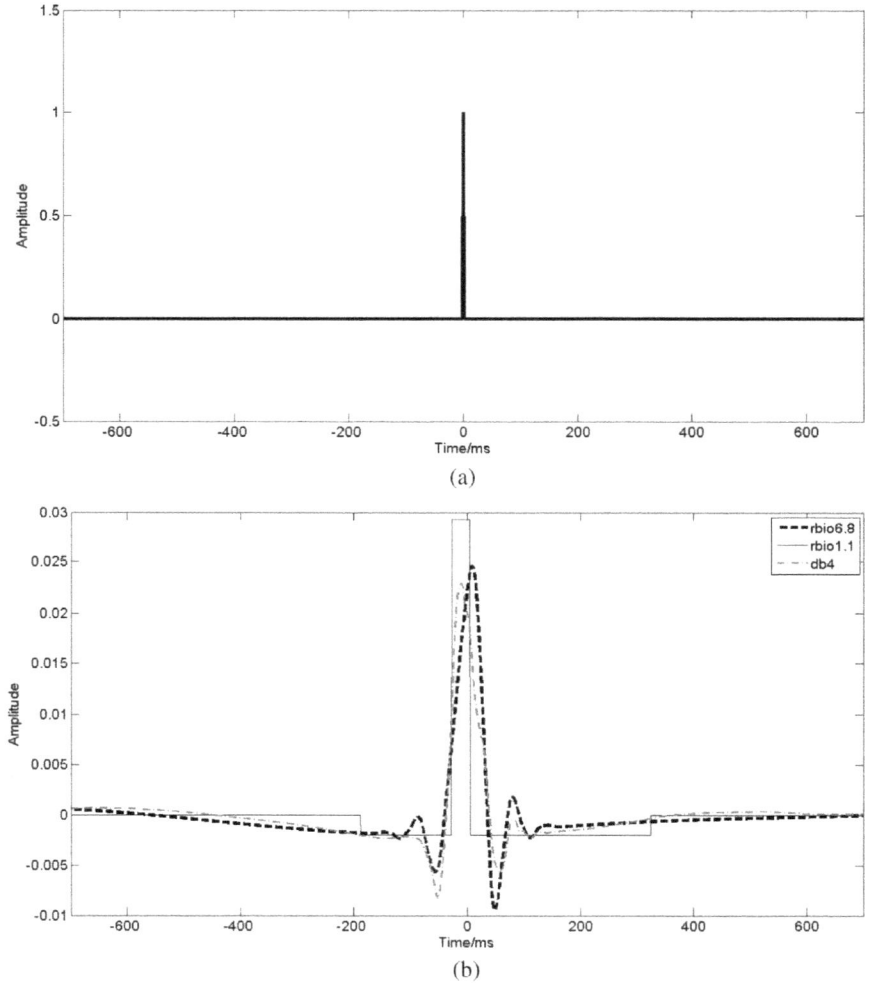

Figure 2.9 Examples of the impulse responses of the wavelet filters (the coefficients at several levels are used for the signal reconstruction). (a) Unit impulse. (b) Impulse response. The duration of the unit impulse is 1400 ms (−700 to 700 ms). The sampling frequency of the unit impulse is 1000 Hz, and the number of levels for the decomposition is 10 according to Eq. (2-11). The coefficients at levels #9, #8, #7, and #6 are used for signal reconstruction.

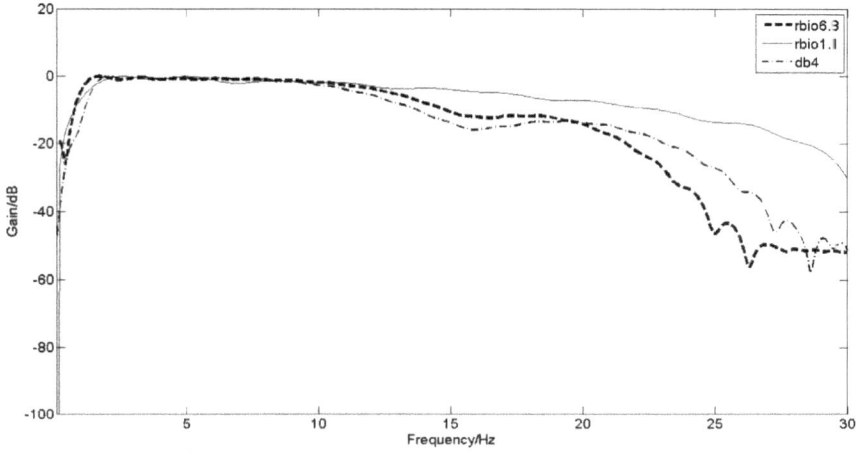

(a)

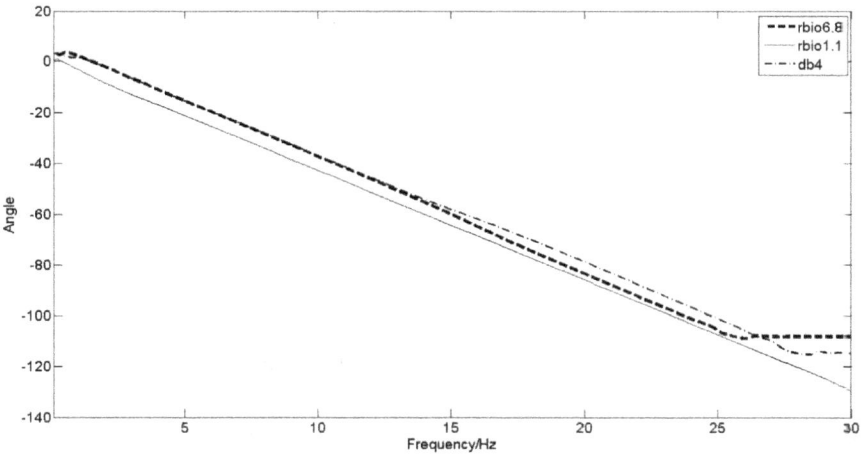

(b)

Figure 2.10 Examples of the magnitude responses of the wavelet filters (the coefficients at several levels are used for the signal reconstruction). (a) Magnitude response. (b) Phase response. The duration of the unit impulse is 1400 ms (−700 to 700 ms). The sampling frequency of the unit impulse is 1000 Hz, and the number of levels for the decomposition is 10 according to Eq. (2-11). The coefficients at levels #9, #8, #7, and #6 are used for the signal reconstruction.

is inappropriate for continuous ERP data. Figure 2.10 shows the magnitude and phase responses of the frequency responses of the three wavelet filters shown in Figure 2.9. The frequency responses shown in Figure 2.10 are the DFTs of the impulse responses. On the basis of the phase responses, choosing between the Daubechies wavelet "db4" and the reverse biorthogonal wavelet "rbio6.8" is difficult. From the magnitude responses, we decide to choose "rbio6.8" for one key reason. The magnitude response of the wavelet filter using "rbio6.8" starts attenuating from approximately 1.5 Hz but that using "db4" starts attenuating from 2 Hz. ERPs can have a very low frequency. Therefore, choosing "rbio6.8" for the wavelet filter would be more appropriate. In fact, without employing the impulse response of the wavelet filter using "rbio1.1," we are able to reject it in terms of the magnitude response for the same reason as that when "db4" is used.

After investigating over 100 wavelets in our previous study (Cong *et al.*, 2012), we found that "rbio6.8" is the best choice for filtering the ERP data. This wavelet has also been used in another study (Astikainen Cong, Ristaniemi, & Hietanen, 2013) to filter ERPs.

We should note that the magnitude response starts attenuating from approximately 10 Hz. According to this wavelet filter property, the spontaneous activity can be removed to some extent.

2.6.8 *Effect of sampling frequency on the wavelet filter*

In the wavelet design, the effect of the sampling frequency was previously ignored. In terms of the DWT implementation shown in Figure 2.6, the number of levels of the wavelet decomposition can be different when the sampling frequencies are different, which is also clearly defined by Eq. (2-11). Figures 2.11 and 2.12 respectively show the impulse responses and frequency responses of the wavelet and DFT filters under different sampling frequencies of the input signals. Obviously, the sampling frequency does not affect the DFT filter but affects the wavelet filter. In practice, collecting ERP data using a higher sampling frequency is prudent, which allows choosing the most appropriate sampling frequency in the wavelet filter design.

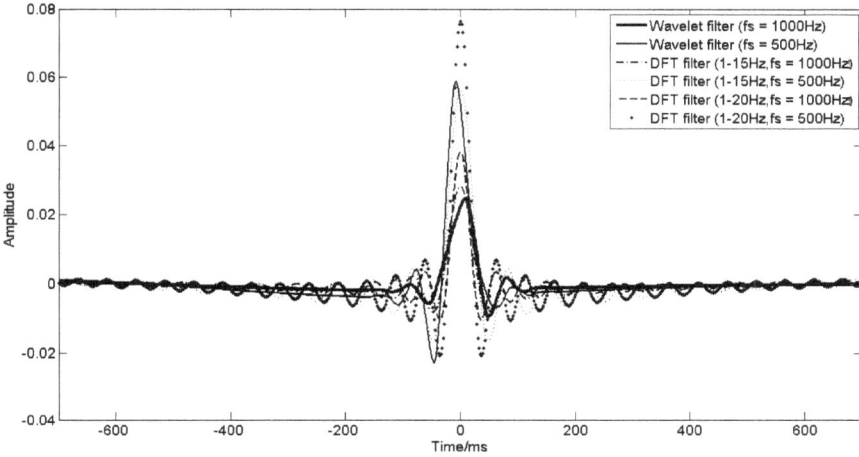

Figure 2.11 Impulse responses of the wavelet and DFT filters under different input signal sampling frequencies. The duration of the unit impulse is 1400 ms (-700 to 700 ms). The sampling frequencies of the unit impulse are 1000 and 500 Hz, and the numbers of levels for the decomposition are respectively 10 and 9 according to Eq. (2-11). The coefficients at levels #9, #8, #7, and #6 are used for the signal reconstruction at the 1000-Hz sampling frequency. The coefficients at levels #8, #7, #6, and #5 are used for the signal reconstruction at the 500-Hz sampling frequency. For the DFT, the number of bins is 10 times the sampling frequency.

2.7 Linear Superposition Rule of the Wavelet Filter and Benefit of the Wavelet Filter in Contrast to the Digital Filter

Similar to the digital and DFT filters, the wavelet filter also obeys the linear superposition rule. If wavelet filter f is applied on the averaged EEG data modeled by Eq. (1-2), the wavelet output is expressed as

$$y_m(t) = f[z_m(t)] = \frac{1}{L} \sum_{l=1}^{L} f[z_m(t, l)].$$ (2-12)

Therefore, Eq. (2-12) shows that performing wavelet filtering on the EEG data for each single trial is unnecessary. From Eq. (1-2), the wavelet filter

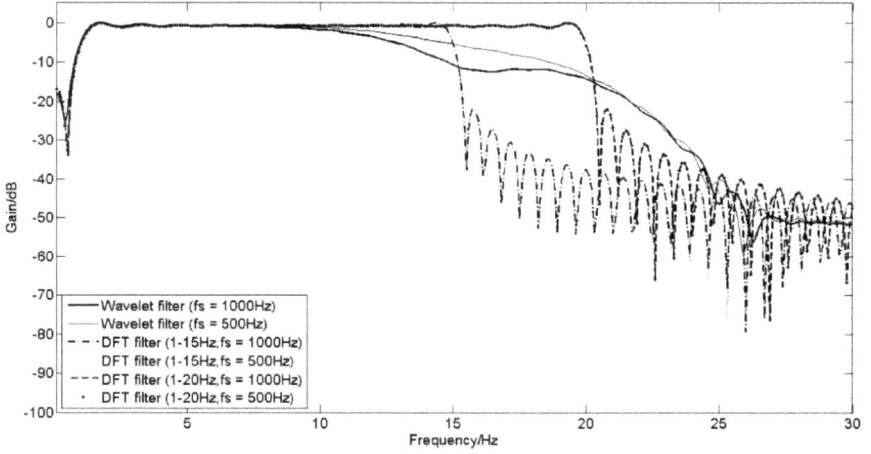

(a)

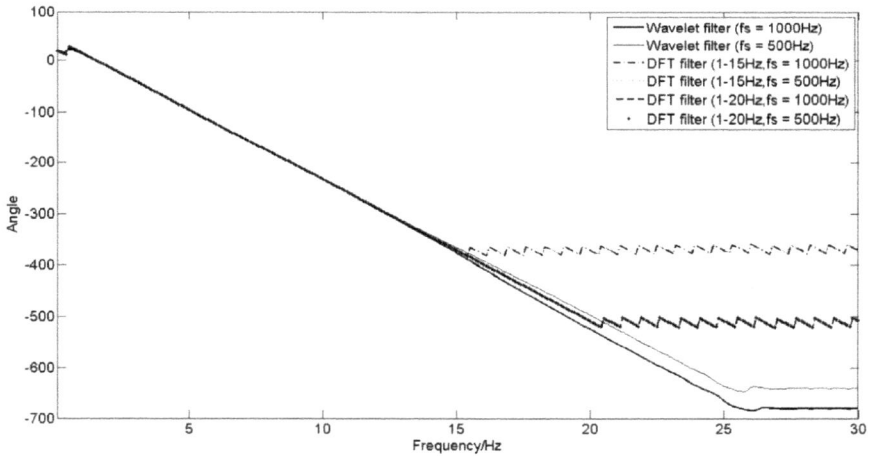

(b)

Figure 2.12   Frequency responses of the wavelet and DFT filters unders different input signal sampling frequencies. (a) Mangitude responses. (b) Phase responses. The duration of the unit impulse is 1400 ms (-700 to 700 ms). The sampling frequencies of the unit impulse are 1000 and 500 Hz, and the filter setup is the same as that shown in Figure 2.11.

output of the averaged EEG data is expressed as

$$y_m(t) = f[z_m(t)]$$

$$= f\left[a_{m,1} \cdot s_1(t) + \cdots + a_{m,r} \cdot s_r(t) + \cdots + a_{m,R} \cdot s_R(t) + v_m(t)\right]$$

$$= f\left[a_{m,1} \cdot s_1(t)\right] + \cdots + f\left[a_{m,r} \cdot s_r(t)\right] + \cdots + f\left[a_{m,R} \cdot s_R(t)\right]$$

$$+ f\left[v_m(t)\right]$$

$$= a_{m,1} \cdot f\left[s_1(t)\right] + \cdots + a_{m,r} \cdot f[s_r(t)] + \cdots + a_{m,R} \cdot f[s_R(t)]$$

$$+ f[v_m(t)]. \tag{2-13}$$

In Eq. (2-13), the EEG sources whose frequency contents are outside the pass band of the wavelet filter shown in Figure 2.12 can be rejected, and those whose frequency contents over 10 Hz and below 1.5 Hz can be partially removed. As a result, the wavelet filter can assist in reducing the number of sources in the EEG data and in improving the signal-to-noise ratio (SNR) of the EEG data (Cong *et al.*, 2011). In the next section, we will show examples of these positive effects.

2.8 Comparison Between the Wavelet and Digital Filters: Case Study on the Waveform and Magnitude Spectrum

In this section, we show an example of filtering ordinarily averaged EEG data (ERP data) using the wavelet and digital filters. The frequency responses of the two filters are shown in Figure 2.12. Before the averaging process, EEG data preprocessing has been applied to remove the artifacts. Figure 2.13 shows the waveforms and magnitude spectrum. Obviously, the wavelet filter removes more frequency contents in the low frequency (below 1 Hz), which greatly assists the filtering in the low-frequency drift while maintaining the low-frequency content of the ERPs.

In particular, the waveform filtered by the wavelet filter becomes smoother. This result indicates that the high-frequency contents of the ordinarily averaged waveform have been partially removed, which is also observed in the magnitude spectrum. We will show the positive effect of the wavelet filter relative to this point in the next section.

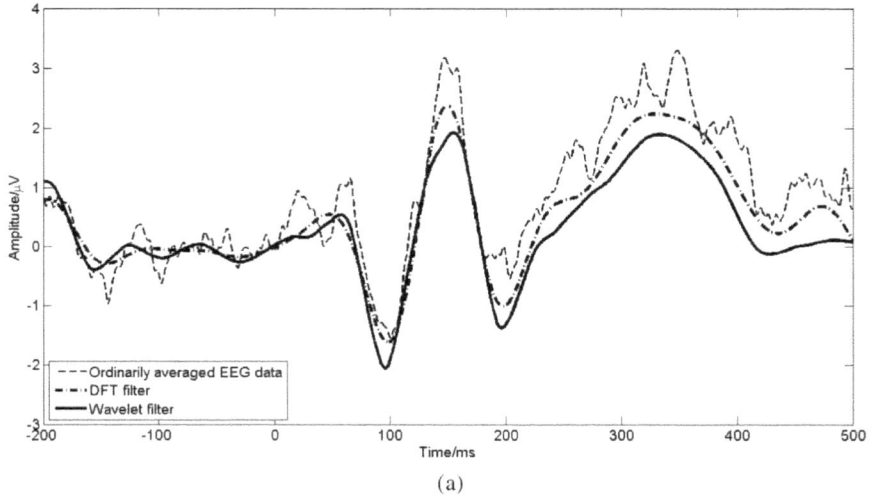

(a)

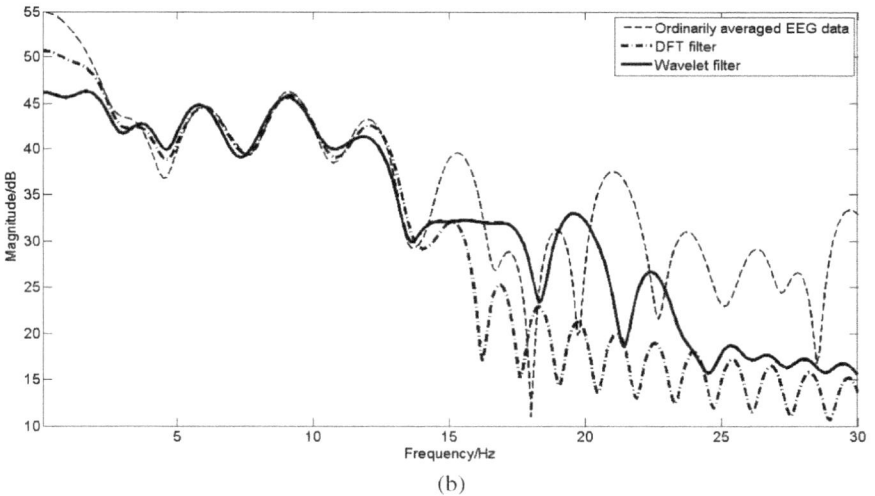

(b)

Figure 2.13　Waveforms and magnitude spectra of the ordinarily averaged EEG and filtered data. The sampling frequency is 1000 Hz. For the wavelet filter, wavelet "ribio6.8" is used. The number of levels for the decomposition is 10 according to Eq. (2-11), and the coefficients at levels #9, #8, #7, and #6 are used for the signal reconstruction. For the DFT filter, the number of bins is 10 times the sampling frequency, and the pass band is from 1 to 15 Hz.

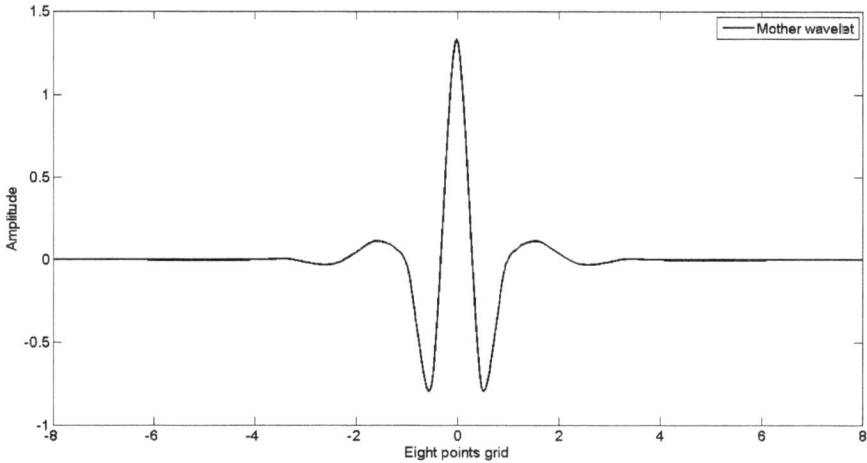

Figure 2.14   Mother wavelet of the reverse biorthogonal wavelet with a 6.8 order.

2.9 Recommendation for the Wavelet Filter Design

We recommend using the reverse biorthogonal wavelet with order 6.8 to design a satisfactory wavelet filter. Figure 2.14 shows its mother wavelet.

Specifically, when the sampling frequencies are 1000, 500, and 250 Hz, the numbers of levels for the wavelet decomposition are 10, 9, and 8, respectively, and the detail coefficients of the number of levels for the signal reconstruction are at levels #9, #8, #7, and #6; levels #8, #7, #6, and #5; and levels #7, #6, #5 and #4, respectively.

2.10 Summary: ERP Data Processing Approach Using DFT or Wavelet Filter

The advantage of the DFT and wavelet filters over the FIR and IIR filters is that the former are effective in filtering EEG data with a one-epoch duration in ERP experiments. They have been used to study the mismatch negativity (MMN) in a continuous paradigm (Cong *et al.*, 2012; Kalyakin *et al.*, 2007).

The ERP data processing approach based on the DFT or wavelet filter includes three steps as follows:

(1) Preprocessing of single-trial EEG data to remove the artifacts.
(2) Averaging the EEG data over single trials.

(3) Applying the DFT or wavelet filter to the averaged EEG data.

In particular, we suggest that single trials that contain artifacts should be discarded, and no digital filter should be used in the first step.

2.11 Existing Key Problem and Potential Solution

Section 2.5.4 presented that only the approximation coefficients are decomposed in the DWT. Thus, division of the narrower bands to filter the averaged EEG data is not allowed. In reality, both approximation and detail coefficients are decomposed in the wavelet packet decomposition. When the latter is decomposed, we can expect a more precise wavelet filter design in terms of the filter's frequency response and spectral properties of the ERP.

2.12 MATLAB Codes

2.12.1 *DFT filter function*

function y = f_filterFFT(x,M,fs,freqLowCut,freqHighCut)

%% x: input signal

%% M : number of points for DFT/FFT

%% fs: sampling frequency of the signal

%% freqLowCut: low cutoff frequency of the filter

%% freqHighCut: high cutoff frequency of the filter

%% y: output of the filter

freqBin = fs/M;%% frequency represented by one frequency bin

%% parameters for FFT-filter

binLowCut = ceil(freqLowCut/freqBin);%% the frequency bin corresponds to the low frequency

binHighCut = ceil(freqHighCut/freqBin); %% the frequency bin corresponds to the high frequency

binLowCut2 = (M/2+1)+(M/2+1-binLowCut);%% the frequency bin corresponds to the low frequency binHighCut2 = (M/2+1)+(M/2+1-binHighCut); %% the frequency bin corresponds to the high frequency

%% M-point DFT

%%%% signal is length - N

X = fft(x,M);

Z = zeros(M,1);

Z(binLowCut:binHighCut) = X(binLowCut:binHighCut);

Z(binHighCut2:binLowCut2) = X(binHighCut2:binLowCut2);

z = ifft(Z,M);

y = z(1:length(x));

2.12.2 *Wavelet filter function*

%%% This code was written by Dr. Yixiang Huang (jetload@126.com)

function y = f_filterWavelet(x,lv,wname,KP)

%% x: input signal

%% lv: number of levels for wavelet decomposition

%% wname: name of wavelet for wavelet filter

%% KP: numbers of the levels of selected coefficients for reconstruction

%% y: output of the filter

%% Note: wavelet toolbox of MATLAB is needed

kp = (lv+2)*ones(size(KP))-KP;

[c l]=wavedec(x,lv,wname);

k = length(kp);

c2=zeros(size(c));

a=0;

b=0;

```
for i=1:k
  if kp(i) == 1
        a=1;
        b=l(1);
      else

    a=0;
        b=0;
        for j=1:kp(i)
          a=b;
          b=b+l(j);
        end
  end
        c2(a:b)=c(a:b);
end
y = waverec(c2,l,wname);
```

2.12.3 *Frequency responses of DFT filter and wavelet filter*

```
clear;
clc;
close all;
tic
%%
NumSamps = 700;
fs = 1000;
Dura = 1000*ceil(NumSamps/fs);
FFTNumSamps=fs*10;
```

```
freqRs=fs/FFTNumSamps;

freqLow=fs/FFTNumSamps;

freqHigh=30;

binLow=freqLow/freqRs;

binHigh=freqHigh/freqRs;

timeIndex=(1:(2*NumSamps-1))*1000/fs;

freqIndex=freqLow:freqRs:freqHigh;

sig=[zeros(NumSamps-1,1);1; zeros(NumSamps-1,1)];

tIndex = linspace(-Dura,Dura,length(sig));

%%%%%%%%%%%%%%%%%%%%% DFT filter

DFfreqLow=1;

DFfreqHigh=15;

DFsig=f_filterFFT(sig,FFTNumSamps,fs,DFfreqLow,DFfreqHigh);

DFsigFFT=fft(DFsig,FFTNumSamps);

spec=abs(DFsigFFT(binLow:binHigh,:));

DFfreqResp=20*log10(spec/max(spec));

DFphase = 2*pi* phase(DFsigFFT(binLow:binHigh));%% phase

%%%%%%%%%%%%%%%%%%%%% Wavelet Filter

lv=10;

wname=[ 'rbio6.8'];

KP=[9 8 7 6];

WAVELETsig=f_filterWavelet(sig,lv,wname,KP);

WAVELETsigFFT=fft(WAVELETsig,FFTNumSamps);

spec=abs(WAVELETsigFFT(binLow:binHigh,:));

WAVELETfreqResp=20*log10(spec/max(spec));

WAVELETphase = 2*pi*phase(WAVELETsigFFT(binLow:binHigh));
```

```
%%
figure
set(gcf, 'outerposition',get(0, 'screensize'))
axes( 'fontsize',14)
h=plot(tIndex,DFsig, 'r-.');
set(h, 'linewidth',2)
hold on
h=plot(tIndex,WAVELETsig, 'k–');
set(h, 'linewidth',2)
xlim([min(tIndex) max(tIndex)])
titleName=[ 'Impulse Response of Unit Impulse'];
title(titleName)
xlabel( 'Time/ms', 'fontsize',14)
ylabel( 'Amplitude')
grid on
legend( 'DFT filter', 'Wavelet filter')
%%
figure
set(gcf, 'outerposition',get(0, 'screensize'))
axes( 'fontsize',14)
h=plot(freqIndex,DFfreqResp, 'r-.');
set(h, 'linewidth',2)
hold on
h=plot(freqIndex,WAVELETfreqResp, 'k–');
set(h, 'linewidth',2)
xlim([freqLow freqHigh])
```

```
ylim([-100 5])
titleName=['Magnitude responses of frequency responses for different filters'];
title(titleName)
xlabel('Frequency/Hz','fontsize',14)
ylabel('Attenuation/dB')
grid on
legend('DFT filter','Wavelet filter','location','southwest')
%%
figure
set(gcf,'outerposition',get(0,'screensize'))
axes('fontsize',14)
h=plot(freqIndex,DFphase,'r-.');
set(h,'linewidth',2)
hold on
h=plot(freqIndex,WAVELETphase,'k-');
set(h,'linewidth',2)
xlim([freqLow freqHigh])
titName=['Phase responses of different filters'];
title(titName)
xlabel('Frequency/Hz','fontsize',14)
ylabel('Angle/degree')
grid on
legend('DFT filter','Wavelet filter')
%%
toc
```

References

Adeli, H., Zhou, Z., & Dadmehr, N. (2003). Analysis of EEG records in an epileptic patient using wavelet transform. *Journal of Neuroscience Methods*, *123*(1), 69–87.

Astikainen, P., Cong, F., Ristaniemi, T. & Hietanen, J. K. (2013). Event-related potentials to unattended changes in facial expressions: Detection of regularity violations or encoding of emotions? *Frontiers in Human Neuroscience*, *7*, 557. doi: 10.3389/fnhum.2013.00557.

Atienza, M., Cantero, J. L. & Quian Quiroga, R. (2005). Precise timing accounts for posttraining sleep-dependent enhancements of the auditory mismatch negativity. *NeuroImage, 26*(2), 628–634. doi: 10.1016/j.neuroimage.2005.02.014.

Berger, H. (1929). Ueber das Elektrenkephalogramm des Menschen. *Archives fur Psychiatrie Nervenkrankheiten*, *87*, 527–570.

Bostanov, V. & Kotchoubey, B. (2006). The t-CWT: A new ERP detection and quantification method based on the continuous wavelet transform and Student's t-statistics. *Clinical Neurophysiology: Official Journal of the International Federation of Clinical Neurophysiology*, *117*(12), 2627–2644. doi: 10.1016/j.clinph.2006.08.012.

Burger, M., Hoppe, U., Kummer, P., Lohscheller, J., Eysholdt, U. & Dollinger, M. (2007). Wavelet-based analysis of MMN responses in children. *Biomedizinische Technik. Biomedical Engineering*, *52*(1), 111–116. doi: 10.1515/BMT.2007.021.

Cohen, M. X. (2014). *Analyzing Neural Time Series Data: Theory and Practice.* Cambridge, MA: The MIT Press.

Coifman, R. R. & Wickerhauser, M. V. (1992). Entropy-based algorithms for best basis selection. *IEEE Transactions on Information Theory*, *38*(2), 713–718.

Cong, F., Huang, Y., Kalyakin, I., Li, H., Huttunen-Scott, T., Lyytinen, H. & Ristaniemi, T. (2012). Frequency response based wavelet decomposition to extract children's mismatch negativity elicited by uninterrupted sound. *Journal of Medical and Biological Engineering*, *32*(3), 205–214.

Cong, F., Leppänen, P. H., Astikainen, P., Hämäläinen, J., Hietanen, J. K. & Ristaniemi, T. (2011). Dimension reduction: Additional benefit of an optimal filter for independent component analysis to extract event-related potentials. *Journal of Neuroscience Methods*, *201*(1), 269–280. doi: 10.1016/j.jneumeth.2011.07.015.

Daubechies, I. (1992). *Ten Lectures on Wavelets.* Society for Industrial and Applied Mathematics.

Donoho, D. L. & Johnstone, I. M. (1994). Ideal denoising in an orthonormal basis chosen from a library of bases. *Comptes Rendus de l'Académie des sciences — Series I, 319*, 1317–1322.

Freeman, W. J. & Quian Quiroga, R. (2013). *Imaging Brain Function With EEG: Advanced Temporal and Spatial Analysis of Electroencephalographic Signals.* New York, NY: Springer.

Jongsma, M. L., Eichele, T., Van Rijn, C. M., Coenen, A. M., Hugdahl, K., Nordby, H. & Quiroga, R. Q. (2006). Tracking pattern learning with single-trial event-related potentials. *Clinical Neurophysiology: Official Journal of the International Federation of Clinical Neurophysiology*, *117*(9), 1957–1973. doi: 10.1016/j.clinph.2006.05.012.

Kalyakin, I., Gonzalez, N., Joutsensalo, J., Huttunen, T., Kaartinen, J., & Lyytinen, H. (2007). Optimal digital filtering versus difference waves on the mismatch negativity in an uninterrupted sound paradigm. *Developmental Neuropsychology*, *31*(3), 429–452. doi: 10.1080/87565640701229607.

Luck, S. J. (2005). *An Introduction to the Event-Related Potential Technique*. Cambridge, MA: The MIT Press.

Mallat, S. (1989). A theory for multiresolution signal decomposition: The wavelet representation. *IEEE Transactions on Pattern Analysis and Machine Intelligence*, *11*(7), 674–693.

Mallat, S. (1999). *A Wavelet Tour of Signal Processing* (2nd ed.). San Diego, CA: Academic Press.

Mitra, S. (2005). *Digital Signal Processing: A Computer Based Approach*. New York, NY: McGraw Hill.

Ocak, H. (2009). Automatic detection of epileptic seizures in EEG using discrete wavelet transform and approximate entropy. *Expert Systems with Applications, 36*, 2027–2036.

Quian Quiroga, R. & Garcia, H. (2003). Single-trial event-related potentials with wavelet denoising. *Clinical Neurophysiology: Official Journal of the International Federation of Clinical Neurophysiology*, *114*(2), 376–390.

Tikkanen, P. E. & Sellin, L. C. (1997). *Wavelet and wavelet packet decomposition of RR and RTmax interval time series*. Paper presented at the IEEE/EMBS 1997.

Wang, D., Miao, Q. & Kang, R. (2009). Robust health evaluation of gearbox subject to tooth failure with wavelet decomposition. *Journal of Sound and Vibration*, *324*(3–5), 1141–1157.

Wilson, W. J. (2004). The relationship between the auditory brain-stem response and its reconstructed waveforms following discrete wavelet transformation. *Clinical Neurophysiology: Official Journal of the International Federation of Clinical Neurophysiology*, *115*(5), 1129–1139. doi: 10.1016/j.clinph.2003.11.019.

Chapter 3

Individual-Level ICA to Extract the ERP Components from the Averaged EEG Data

In this chapter, we introduce the classic independent component analysis (ICA) theory, the special ICA theory in event-related potential (ERP) data processing, and the systematic ICA approach to extract the ERP components from the ERP data of only one subject under one condition. We call this ICA application in this book as individual ICA. Here, ERP data denote the averaged electroencephalography (EEG) data over single trials.

3.1 Classic ICA Theory

3.1.1 *Brief history*

The first paper that formally introduced the ICA theory, algorithm, and application appeared in 1994 (Comon, 1994). It was published in a special issue of the Elsevier journal *Signal Processing*. Thereafter, thousands of papers on ICA have been published. By March 2014, over 28,800 and 2400 papers in the Web of Science can be searched when "ICA" is used as the title for the topic and as a keyword, respectively.

Theoretically, ICA is a perfect tool for solving the problem of blind source separation (BSS) (Comon, Jutten, & Herault, 1991; Jutten & Herault, 1991). Since 1999, 10 international conferences with the theme ICA/BSS have been held. In 2001, a very popular textbook was published (Hyvarinen, Karhunen, & Oja, 2001), and in 2010, a handbook on ICA and BSS was released (Comon & Jutten, 2010).

3.1.2 *ICA model, assumptions, and solution in obtaining independent components*

3.1.2.1 *Model*

ICA was developed to specifically solve the cocktail-party problem (Cichocki & Amari, 2003; Comon & Jutten, 2010; Hyvarinen *et al.*, 2001). The problem can be described by a linear transform model.

Figure 3.1 shows an example of the scenario of the BSS problem and a simple illustration of the problem (Shi, 2011). In this example, a person is talking, which is a sound source. Meanwhile, other sources of sound are also present, e.g., the ringing of a phone, airplane noise, etc. Each microphone in the room records the mixture of sounds. This entire process can be expressed as

$$z_m(t) = a_{m,1} \cdot s_1(t) + \cdots + a_{m,r} \cdot s_r(t) + \cdots + a_{m,R} \cdot s_R(t) + v_m(t),$$

$$(3\text{-}1)$$

where
   $z_m(t)$ is the recording by a sensor (e.g., the microphone shown in Figure 3.1);
   m is the number of the sensor; $m = 1, 2, \ldots, M$;
   r is the number of the source; $r = 1, 2, \ldots, R$;
   $s_r(t)$ represents the source (e.g., sound source shown in Figure 3.1);
   $a_{m,r}$ denotes the coefficient between source #r and the point where sensor #m is located in space; and
   $v_m(t)$ is the background noise.

If the power of each sound source is comparable, we can hardly hear a particular sound of interest. This problem is not new. In this case, a technical solution to clearly hear a particular source is to extract the source from the mixture or separate the mixture into individual sources. In the model, however, the sources are unknown, as well as the coefficient between any source and any sensor. Thus, resolving the problem is very difficult. After ICA was developed, the problem becomes theoretically solvable (Cichocki & Amari, 2003; Comon & Jutten, 2010; Hyvarinen *et al.*, 2001). For simplicity, we do not provide the theoretical details in resolving this problem in this book. We only present the key solution.

(a)

(b)

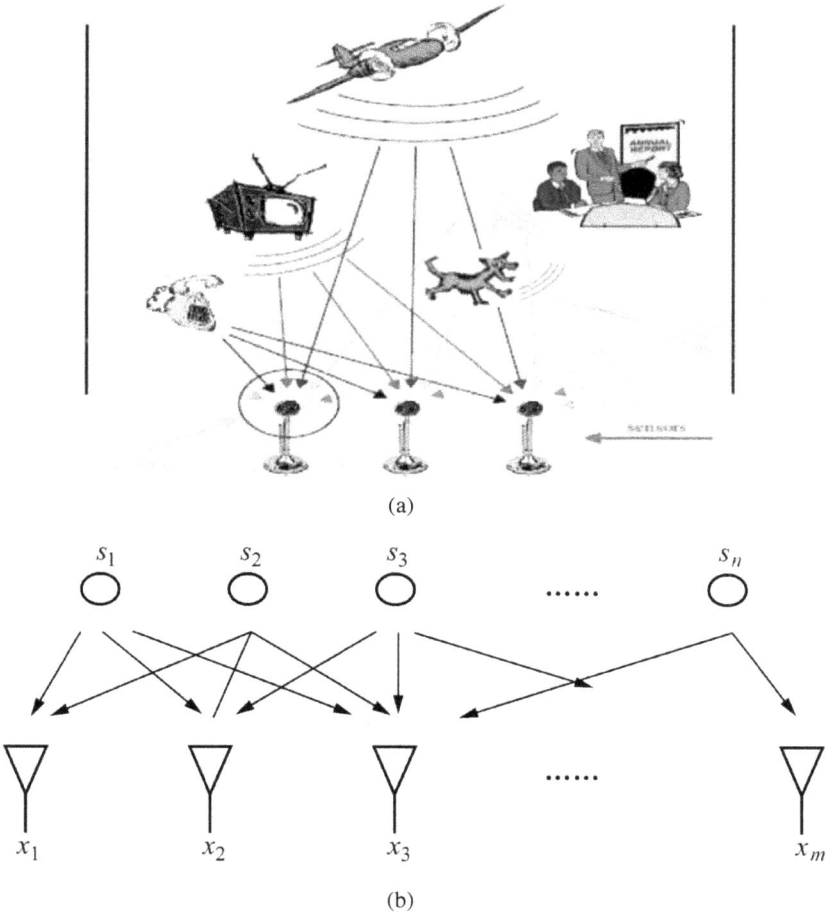

Figure 3.1 (a) Scenario of a BSS problem (adapted from the Internet). (b) Simple illustration of the problem. This example is the instantaneous model, which means that no sound reflection is present, and any sound source in the room has no delay. This condition is not possible in a normal office room. In practice, the convolutive model is considered (Comon & Jutten, 2010), which is not included in this book.

Equation (3-1) is called the noisy linear transform model. In the basic ICA model (Cichocki & Amari, 2003; Comon & Jutten, 2010; Hyvarinen *et al.*, 2001), no additive noise is present; the noise-free model is expressed as

$$x_m(t) = a_{m,1} \cdot s_1(t) + \cdots + a_{m,r} \cdot s_r(t) + \cdots + a_{m,R} \cdot s_R(t). \qquad (3\text{-}2)$$

In matrix-vector form, the model is written as

$$\mathbf{x}(t) = \mathcal{A}\mathbf{s}(t), \tag{3-3}$$

where $\mathbf{x}(t) = [x_1(t), x_2(t), \ldots, x_M(t)]^T \in \mathfrak{R}^{M \times 1}$ is the observation vector, $\mathcal{A} \in \mathfrak{R}^{M \times R}$ represents the mixing matrix, and $\mathbf{s}(t) = [s_1(t), s_2(t), \ldots, s_R(t)]^T \in \mathfrak{R}^{R \times 1}$ denotes the source vector.

3.1.2.2 *Classification of the ICA models*

The ICA models can be classified into three groups.

(1) When the number of sensors is larger than the number of sources ($M > R$), the model is over-determined.
(2) When the number of sensors is equal to the number of sources ($M = R$), the model is determined.
(3) When the number of sensors is smaller than the number of sources ($M < R$), the model is under-determined.

3.1.2.3 *Assumptions*

In order to perform the ICA to separate the mixture $x_m(t)$ in Eq. (3-2) into independent components, three fundamental assumptions (Cichocki & Amari, 2003; Comon & Jutten, 2010; Hyvarinen *et al.*, 2001) are made.

(1) Mixing matrix $\mathcal{A}$ is full rank.
(2) At most, one source with a Gaussian distribution is present.
(3) The sources are statistically independent from one another.

3.1.2.4 *Solution*

After one unmixing matrix is learned from the mixture $\mathbf{x}(t)$, the independent components can be expressed as

$$y_r(t) = w_{r,1} \cdot x_1(t) + \cdots + w_{r,m} \cdot x_m(t) + \cdots + w_{r,M} \cdot x_M(t) \tag{3-4}$$

$$\mathbf{y}(t) = \mathbf{W}\mathbf{x}(t), \tag{3-5}$$

where $\mathbf{y}(t) = [y_1(t), y_2(t), \ldots, y_R(t)]^T \in \Re^{R \times 1}$ represents the independent component vector and $\mathbf{W} \in \Re^{R \times M}$ is the unmixing matrix. For a perfect ICA solution, one independent component is associated with only one source.

Obviously, the solution is very simple after the unmixing matrix is successfully estimated by the ICA algorithm.

3.1.3 *ICA algorithm and indeterminacies of independent components*

3.1.3.1 *Classification of ICA algorithms based on the ICA models*

As mentioned earlier, the ICA models can be divided into three categories. Therefore, the ICA algorithms for different models can be different. Irrespective of which algorithm is used, the number of extracted ICA components is the same as the number of sources.

Before the ICA, the over-determined model is usually converted into a determined model (Cichocki & Amari, 2003; Comon & Jutten, 2010; Hyvarinen *et al.*, 2001). Then, for both the over-determined and determined models, the determined ICA algorithm should be used.

For the under-determined ICA model, the under-determined ICA algorithm should be used. This type of ICA algorithm is not considered in this book.

3.1.3.2 *ICA algorithm for the determined model*

The determined ICA model is given as

$$\mathbf{x}(t) = \mathbf{As}(t), \tag{3-6}$$

where $\mathbf{x}(t) = [x_1(t), x_2(t), \ldots, x_R(t)]^T \in \Re^{R \times 1}$ represents the observation vector and $\mathbf{A} \in \Re^{R \times R}$ is the mixing matrix, which is a square matrix.

Then, using the ICA algorithm, we obtain the unmixing matrix $\mathbf{W} \in \Re^{R \times R}$ to produce the ICA components using the following equation:

$$\mathbf{y}(t) = \mathbf{Wx}(t). \tag{3-7}$$

Many theories have been proposed to obtain the unmixing matrix (Cichocki & Amari, 2003; Comon & Jutten, 2010; Hyvarinen *et al.*, 2001).

Most ICA algorithms are iterative. We choose one iterative algorithm (based on the information theory) for illustration as follows:

$$\mathbf{W}(i + 1) = \mathbf{W}(i) + \mu \left\{ \mathbf{I} + \varphi \left[\mathbf{y}_i(t) \right] \mathbf{y}_i(t)^T \right\} \mathbf{W}(i) \qquad (3\text{-}8)$$

$$\mathbf{y}_i(t) = \mathbf{W}(i)\mathbf{x}(t), \qquad (3\text{-}9)$$

where i denotes the number of iteration, μ is the learning step and is usually a small number, φ is a nonlinear function (which is related to the probability density functions of the sources), and $\mathbf{y}_i(t)$ represents the component vector obtained at the ith iteration.

3.1.3.3 *Implementation of the ICA algorithm*

The first step of the iterative ICA algorithm is to initialize the unmixing matrix. The most frequently used method is the random generation of an unmixing matrix for $\mathbf{W}(1)$.

Then, $\mathbf{W}(2)$ is derived according to Eqs. (3-8) and (3-9). Next, the difference between $\mathbf{W}(2)$ and $\mathbf{W}(1)$ is calculated. If the difference is smaller than a predefined threshold, the iteration stops, and $\mathbf{W} = \mathbf{W}(2)$. Otherwise, $\mathbf{W}(3)$ is derived.

The iteration process continues until the difference between $\mathbf{W}(i + 1)$ and $\mathbf{W}(i)$ is small enough or the predefined number of iterations is achieved. In the first case, we consider that the ICA algorithm converges to a stationary point. In the second case, the ICA algorithm does not converge.

3.1.3.4 *Definitions of the global and local optimization of ICA*

By considering Eq. (3-6), Eq. (3-7) can be written as

$$\mathbf{y}(t) = \mathbf{W}\mathbf{x}(t) = \mathbf{W}\mathbf{A}\mathbf{s}(t) = \mathbf{C}\mathbf{s}(t) \qquad (3\text{-}10)$$

$$\mathbf{C} = \mathbf{W}\mathbf{A} \qquad (3\text{-}11)$$

$$y_r(t) = c_{r,1} \cdot s_1(t) + \cdots + c_{r,r} \cdot s_r(t) + \cdots + c_{r,R} \cdot s_R(t), \quad (3\text{-}12)$$

where $\mathbf{C}$ is called the global matrix (Cichocki & Amari, 2003) and $c_{r,q}$ is the (r, q) element of $\mathbf{C}$ at the rth row and qth column.

Next, we define the two ICA optimization categories in this book.

[Definition: Global optimization]

If only one nonzero element exists in each row and each column of the global matrix, the optimization of the ICA algorithm is defined as global optimization in this book.

This definition suggests that the ICA algorithm converges to the globally optimized point. In such condition, Eq. (3-12) becomes

$$y_r(t) = c_{r,k} \cdot s_k(t), \tag{3-13}$$

where r can be equal or not equal to k. We should note that many global matrices are available that satisfy the global optimization condition. Therefore, under global optimization, both the global and unmixing matrices are not unique.

[Definition: Local optimization]

If at least two nonzero elements exist in one row or one column of the global matrix, the optimization of the ICA algorithm is defined as local optimization in this book.

This definition suggests that the ICA algorithm converges to the locally optimized point. In this case, at least two elements of the global matrix in Eq. (3-12) are not zero, which means that an independent component may still be a mixture of some sources.

3.1.3.5 *Indeterminacies of the independent components*

The independent components have two types of inherent indeterminacies in the variance and polarity of any independent component and the order of all independent components. The polarity of a component is not often mentioned.

Under global optimization, the $c_{r,k}$ value in Eq. (3-13) is not determined because the condition for the global optimization is that only one nonzero element should exist in each row and each column of the global matrix. The magnitude and polarity of $c_{r,k}$ in Eq. (3-13) is not limited. Therefore, the variance in the independent component is also not determined. Equation (3-13) also indicates that the independent component is simply the unknown scaled version of one source.

Figure 3.2 shows four sources (Cong, Kalyakin, Li, *et al.*, 2011) and the simulated mixture of four sensors. This simulation assumes that the number of sensors is equal to the number of sources, i.e., a determined model. Figure 3.3 shows the mixing and unmixing matrices under global optimization. Figure 3.4 shows the extracted components from the mixture [shown in Figure 3.2(b)] when the ICA decomposition is under global optimization. We present two unmixing matrices, both of which satisfy the global optimization condition. For Figure 3.4(a), the unmixing matrix is shown in Figure 3.3(b). For source #2 in Figure 3.2(a), extracted independent components #1 [shown in Figure 3.4(a)] and #2 [shown in Figure 3.4(b)] are the extracted source components. Obviously, the order of the extracted source component can be different from that of the source of interest, which means that the rth independent component in Eq. (3-13) may be associated with the kth source. Furthermore, the variance in the extracted source component can be different from that of the source of interest as well as the polarity of the extracted source component with respect to that of the source of interest.

The variance (including the polarity) and permutation indeterminacies of the ICA components are not considered as problems in some applications, e.g., in speech source separation. However, for ERP data analysis, they should be corrected. In the next section, we demonstrate how the variance and polarity indeterminacies can be corrected.

3.2 ICA Theory in ERP Data Processing: Back Projection

With the development in the ICA research, key issues arise in terms of application requirement (Hyvarinen, 2013). For example, in the ERP data analysis, the variance indeterminacy of the ICA component must be corrected because the ERP amplitude is a very important parameter in ERP data analysis. Therefore, developing the ICA theory to correct the variance indeterminacy of an ICA component has been advocated. Dr. Makeig and his colleagues first reported their research on this subject in 1996 and 1997 (Makeig, Bell, Jung, & Sejnowski, 1996; Makeig, Jung, Bell, Ghahremani, & Sejnowski, 1997). However, until 2011, even little progress has not been made regarding this issue (Cong, Kalyakin, & Ristaniemi, 2011; Cong, Kalyakin, Zheng, & Ristaniemi, 2011).

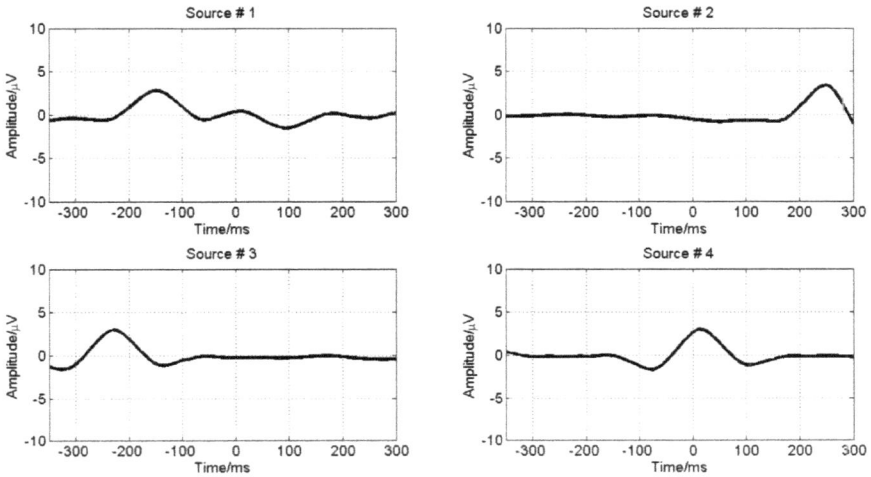

(a)

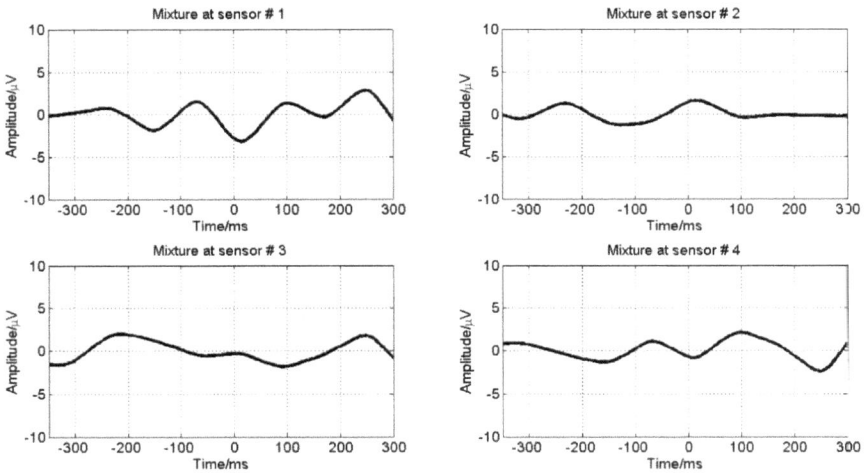

(b)

Figure 3.2 Example of (a) the four sources and (b) simulated mixtures collected by four sensors. The ERP components (extracted by the ICA from the averaged EEG data) are considered as the sources in the simulation, which conform to Eq. (3-6). The mixing matrix (4×4) is randomly generated. The absolute value of the element in the mixing matrix is smaller than one. The mixture is used subsequently for the ICA separation.

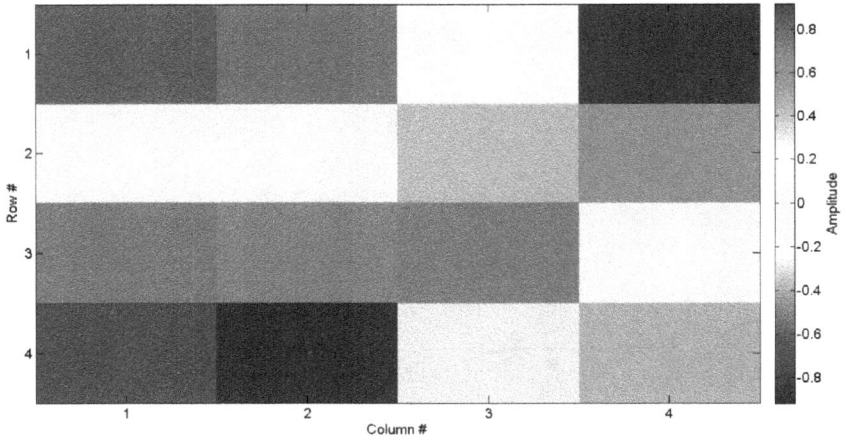

(a)

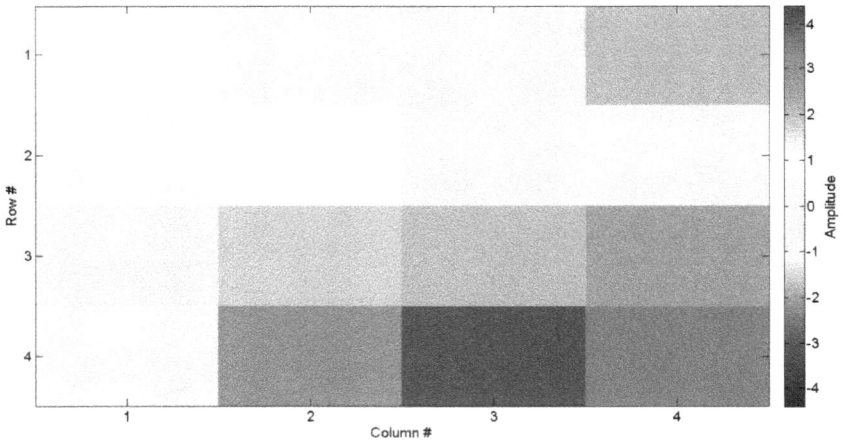

(b)

Figure 3.3   (a) Mixing and (b) unmixing matrices for the ICA decomposition under global optimization.

In the next section, we present the ICA theory to correct the variance and polarity of an independent component.

3.2.1 *Reconsideration of the linear transform model of EEG*

Figure 1.3 shows that a source includes a temporal component and a spatial component (i.e., topography). Both components are equally important.

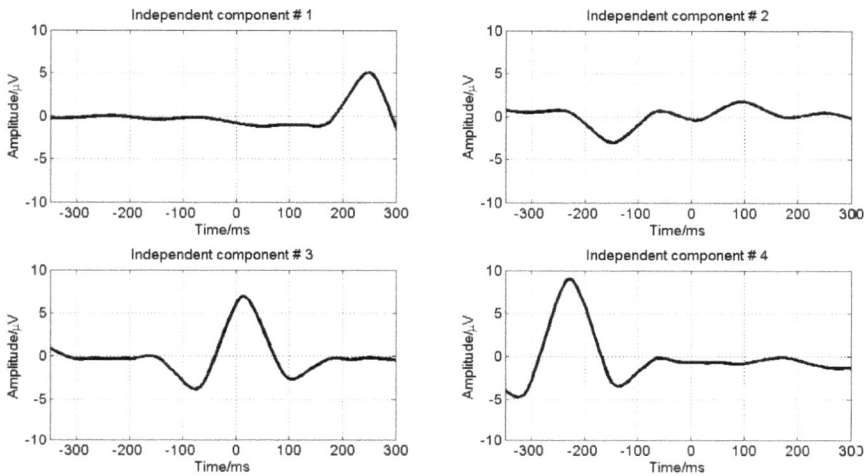

(a)

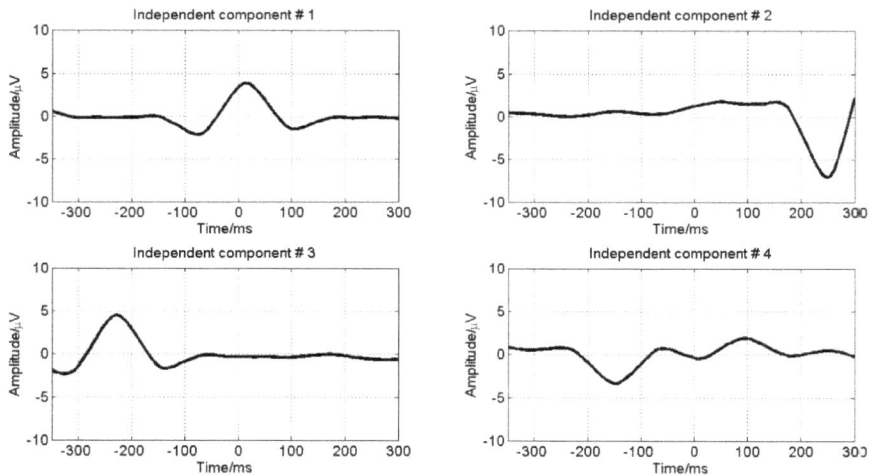

(b)

Figure 3.4 Extracted independent components when the ICA algorithm converges under global optimization. (a) and (b) Two cases with two different unmixing matrices and two different global matrices. The mixtures separated by the ICA algorithm are those shown in Figure 3.2. Because the mixtures are simulated according to Eq. (3-6), we know the sources and the mixing matrix. Therefore, we artificially produce the unmixing matrix under global optimization. This process does not affect the further theoretical analysis.

Following this concept, we write Eq. (3-6) as follows:

$$\mathbf{x}(t) = \mathbf{As}(t) = \mathbf{a}_1 \cdot s_1(t) + \mathbf{a}_2 \cdot s_2(t) + \cdots + \mathbf{a}_R \cdot s_R(t), \qquad (3\text{-}14)$$

where $\mathbf{a}_r \in \mathfrak{R}^{R \times 1}$ denotes the topography shown in Figure 1.3 and is the rth column of $\mathbf{A}$. This expression means that each column of the mixing matrix assumes the topography of one source.

If only one source is present in the brain, Eq. (3-14) is written as

$$\mathbf{x}_r(t) = \mathbf{a}_r \cdot s_r(t) \qquad (3\text{-}15)$$

where $\mathbf{x}_r(t)$ is called the mapping of the rth source along the scalp and $\mathbf{a}_r$ contains the mapping coefficients of the source. In this case, the EEG data in one sensor contain only the scaled version of the source. In other words, the only source is transferred to the point where the sensor is placed along the scalp. In practice, therefore, the EEG data are indeed a mixture of the scaled versions of many sources. The scale of each source is associated with the source topography.

Figure 3.5 shows the simulated EEG data in the case where only one source is present. The only source in the simulated EEG data is source #3 shown in Figure 3.2(a). The simulated data are very neat and only reflect

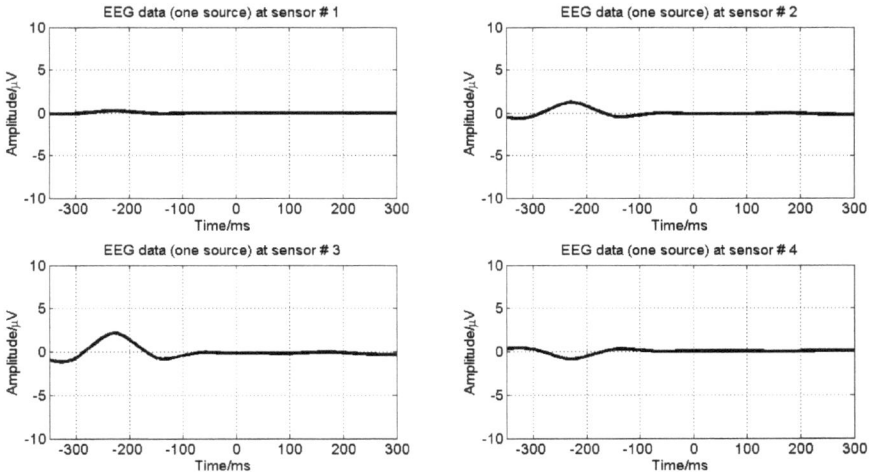

Figure 3.5   Simulated EEG data in the case where only one source exists. The simulation is performed according to Eq. (3-15). The source is #3 shown in Figure 3.2(a).

one type of brain activity. Figure 3.5 shows that the coefficient between the source and the point along the scalp can be different owing to the volume conduction property of the brain (Makeig *et al.*, 1997; Makeig, Westerfield, Jung, *et al.*, 1999; Makeig, Westerfield, Townsend, *et al.*, 1999). For example, after the source is transferred to the point where sensor #1 is located, the scaled source becomes much weaker than the original source. This may be due to the relatively longer distance between the source location in the cortex and the point along the scalp. Moreover, the EEG data polarities at different points can be different. For example, in contrast to the source, they are reversed at the two points where sensors #3 and #4 are located.

Figure 3.6 shows the simulated EEG data in the two cases where two and three sources are present. Figure 3.2(b) shows the simulated data in the case of four sources. Obviously, the EEG data become more complicated with the increase in the number of sources.

We should note that a source is almost invisible at some points along the scalp in contrast to the other sources. For example, source #4 in the EEG data at the point of sensor #3 [shown in Figure 3.6(a)] hardly appears. However, as expressed by Eqs. (3-14) and (3-15), this absence does not mean that source #4 is not transferred to this point. The volume conduction at this point is simply much more reduced in contrast to that at the other points along the scalp. In other words, the scaled version of source #4 is much weaker than those of the other sources at the point of sensor #3, as shown in Figure 3.6(a).

In summary, the EEG data model can be illustrated as follows:

(1) Many sources in the brain are active.
(2) The waveforms of the different sources can peak at different time stamps.
(3) The sources are transferred from their respective locations in the cortex to the points along the scalp, and volume conduction occurs during the transfer.
(4) The degree of volume conduction implicitly generates the scale and polarity distribution, i.e., the topography of the source.
(5) The EEG data collected along the scalp are a mixture of the scaled versions of the sources.

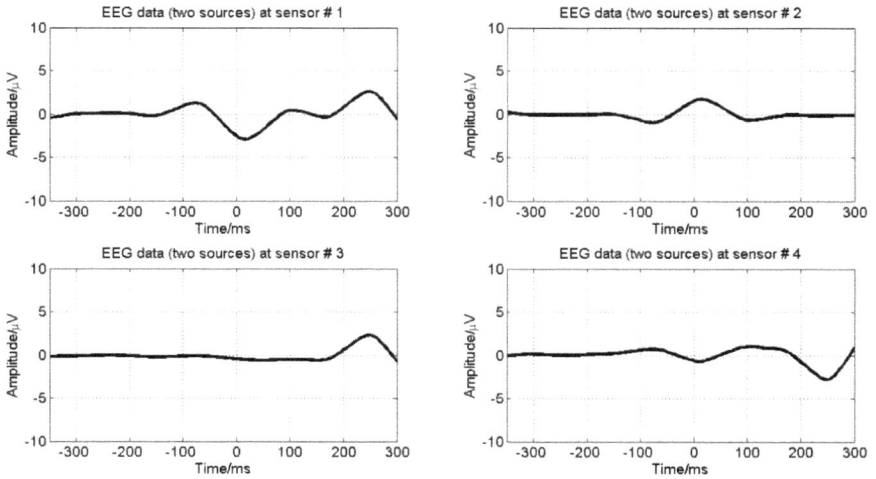

(a)

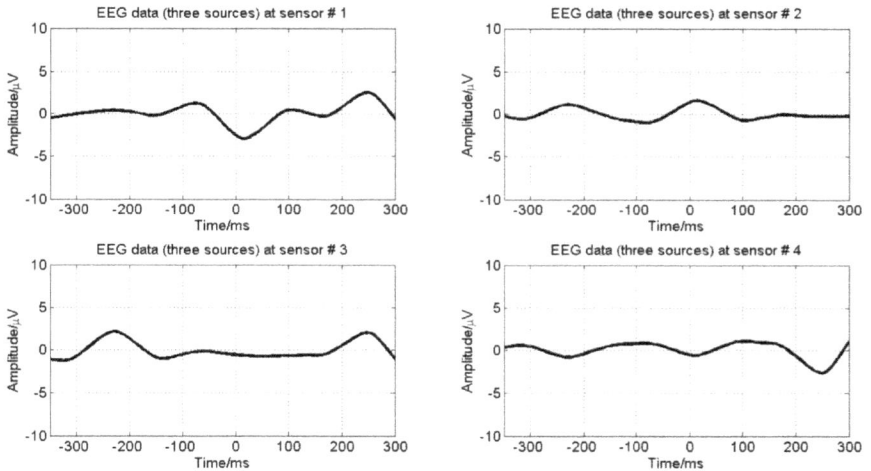

(b)

Figure 3.6   Simulated EEG data in the two cases where two and three sources are present. The simulation is performed according to Eq. (3-14). The two sources in (a) are #2 and #4, as shown in Figure 3.2(a). The three sources in (b) are #2, #3, and #4, as shown in Figure 3.2(a).

3.2.2 *Back-projection of an ICA component to correct the indeterminacies in the variance and polarity*

3.2.2.1 *Introduction to back-projection*

As discussed in Section 3.1.3.5, the variance and polarity of an independent component are not determined. Dr. Makeig and his colleagues suggested projecting an independent component back to the electrode field to correct the indeterminacies of the ICA component. From Eqs. (3-6), (3-14), and (3-7), the back-projection approach (Makeig *et al.*, 1996, 1997) is expressed as follows:

$$\mathbf{e}_q(t) = \mathbf{b}_q \cdot y_q(t) \tag{3-16}$$

$$\mathbf{B} = \mathbf{W}^{-1}, \tag{3-17}$$

where $y_q(t)$ represents the independent component of interest, $\mathbf{B} \in \mathbf{R}^{R \times R}$ is the inverse of unmixing matrix ($\mathbf{W} \in R^{R \times R}$), and $\mathbf{b}_q$ is the qth column of $\mathbf{B}$. In this book, $\mathbf{B}$ is called the back-projection matrix.

We should note that each column in $\mathbf{B}$ contains the topography (i.e., scalp map) of one ICA component. Figure 3.7 shows an example of ICA on the EEG data (Jung, Makeig, Westerfield, *et al.*, 2000). When ICA is applied to extract the ERP component, the ERP component actually

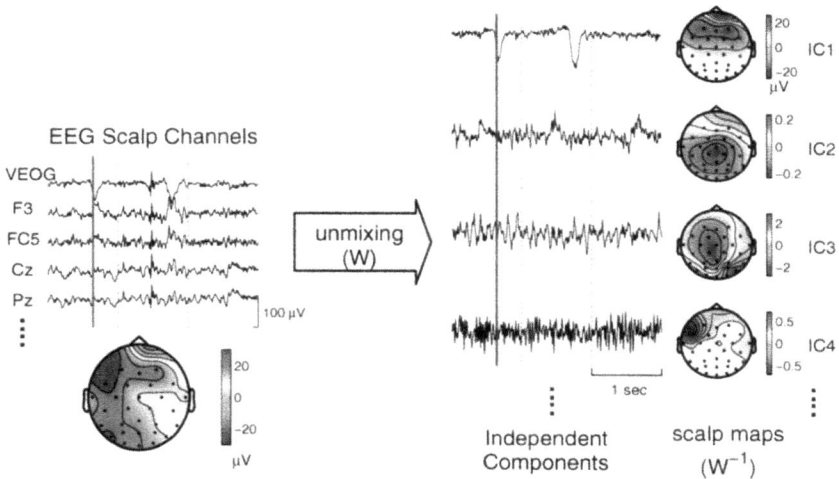

Figure 3.7   Example of the ICA on the EEG data [adapted from Jung *et al.* (2000)].

includes two parts, namely, the temporal independent component and spatial topography.

Furthermore, in terms of the global matrix in Eq. (3-11), the inverse of the unmixing matrix can be expressed as

$$\mathbf{B} = \mathbf{W}^{-1} = \mathbf{A}\mathbf{C}^{-1} = \mathbf{A}\mathcal{C} \qquad (3\text{-}18)$$

$$\mathbf{b}_q = \mathbf{A}\boldsymbol{c}_q, \qquad (3\text{-}19)$$

where $\mathcal{C} = \mathbf{C}^{-1}$ and $\boldsymbol{c}_q$ is the qth column of $\mathcal{C}$.

Obviously, back-projection matrix $\mathbf{B}$ is associated with mixing matrix $\mathbf{A}$. We note that each column of the mixing matrix represents the topography of one source, and each column of the back-projection matrix denotes the topography of one independent component.

However, Eq. (3-16) does not show the difference between the electrode-field EEG data in Eq. (3-16) and the EEG data in Eqs. (3-6) and (3-14). In addition, it does not indicate the association between the back-projection matrix in Eq. (3-17) and the mixing matrix in Eqs. (3-6) and (3-14). Dr. Makeig and his colleagues failed to address this issue. (Makeig *et al.*, 1996, 1997; Makeig, Westerfield, Jung, *et al.*, 1999; Makeig, Westerfield, Townsend, *et al.*, 1999; Onton, Westerfield, Townsend, & Makeig, 2006).

In this book, we introduce the difference and the association according to our previous studies (Cong *et al.*, 2010; Cong, Kalyakin, Li, *et al.*, 2011; Cong, Kalyakin, & Ristaniemi, 2011; Cong, Kalyakin, Zheng, *et al.*, 2011).

3.2.2.2 *Back-projection under global optimization*

Under global optimization, each column and each row of global matrix $\mathbf{C}$ and the inverse of the global matrix, i.e., $\mathcal{C}$, have only one nonzero element. This condition means that $\boldsymbol{c}_q$ has only one nonzero element. Consequently, Eq. (3-19) can be transformed into

$$\mathbf{b}_q = \mathbf{a}_p c_{p,q}, \qquad (3\text{-}20)$$

where $c_{p,q}$ is at the pth row and qth column of $\mathcal{C}$ and is the only nonzero element in the pth row and qth column of $\mathcal{C}$. This equation also indicates that the topography of one independent component under global optimization is simply the scaled version of the mapping coefficients of the corresponding source. Then, after Eq. (3-20) is substituted into Eq. (3-16), the back-projection of one independent component under the global optimization is expressed as

$$\mathbf{e}_q(t) = \mathbf{a}_p \cdot c_{p,q} \cdot y_q(t). \tag{3-21}$$

We should note that $c_{p,q}$ is the only nonzero element in the pth row and qth column of $\mathcal{C}$, and its position is in the pth row and qth column of $\mathcal{C}$. As a result, the only nonzero element in the qth row and pth column of $\mathbf{C}$ is $c_{q,p}$. Moreover, because $\mathcal{C}$ is the inverse of global matrix $\mathbf{C}$

$$c_{p,q} \cdot c_{q,p} = 1. \tag{3-22}$$

Then, according to Eq. (3-13)

$$y_q(t) = c_{q,p} \cdot s_p(t). \tag{3-23}$$

After Eqs. (3-22) and (3-23) are substituted into Eq. (3-21), the back-projection of one independent component under global optimization is expressed as

$$\mathbf{e}_q(t) = \mathbf{a}_p \cdot s_p(t). \tag{3-24}$$

Equation (3-24) indicates that the back-projection of one independent component under global optimization is equal to the mapping of one source, as shown by Eq. (3-15). In this case, although the independent component has variance and polarity indeterminacies, as shown in Figure 3.4, the back-projection of one independent component does not contain any variance and polarity indeterminacies anymore, which is the information presented by Eq. (3-24). This is the reason why back-projection can correct the variance and polarity indeterminacies of one independent component.

Figure 3.8 shows the global matrix and its inverse under global optimization. Obviously, only one nonzero element exists in each row and each column. The two matrices indicate that Eq. (3-22) is valid. Figure 3.9 shows two back-projection matrices under global optimization. According to Eq. (3-20), the column of the back-projection matrix is the scaled version of one column of the mixing matrix. For example, the fourth column in Figure 3.9(a) is the scaled version of the third column

(a)

(b)

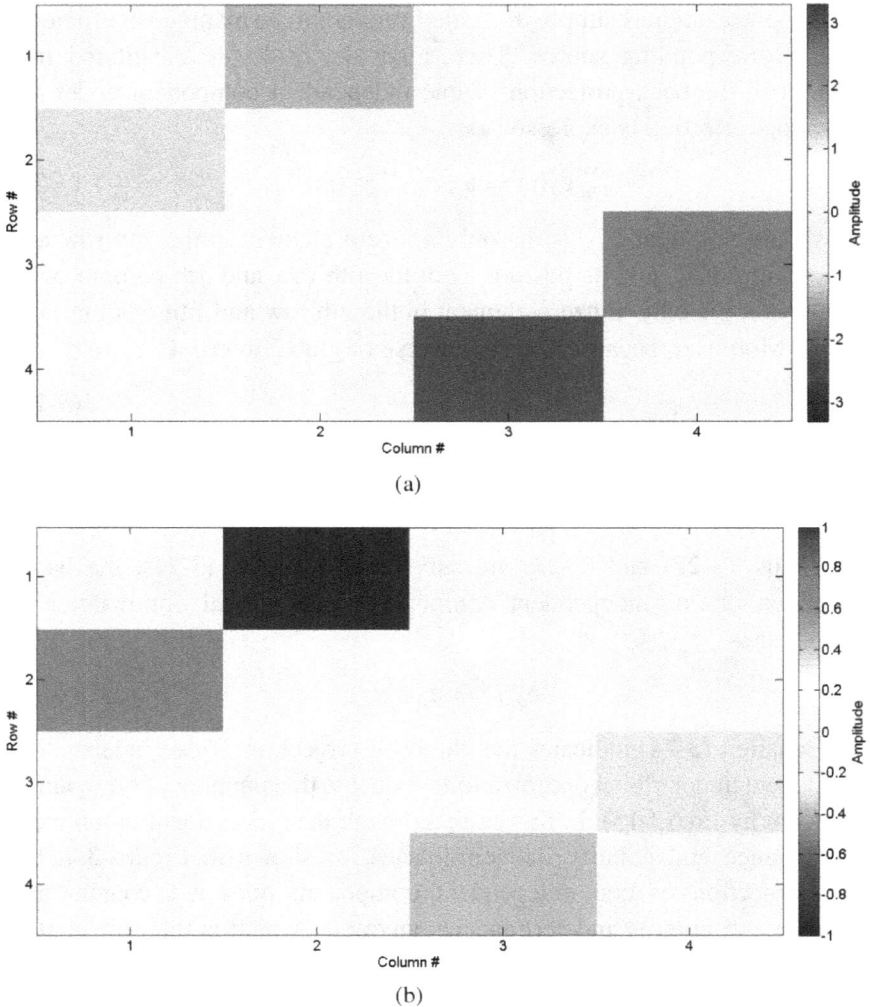

Figure 3.8   (a) Global matrix under global optimization. (b) Inverse of the global matrix in (a). The global matrix is based on the mixing and unmixing matrices shown in Figure 3.3.

of the mixing matrix shown in Figure 3.3(a), and the third column in Figure 3.9(b) is the scaled version of the third column of the mixing matrix shown in Figure 3.3(a). Figure 3.10 shows the back-projection of component #4 in Figure 3.4(a) and the back-projection of component #3 in Figure 3.4(b). Obviously, they are identical because the two unmixing

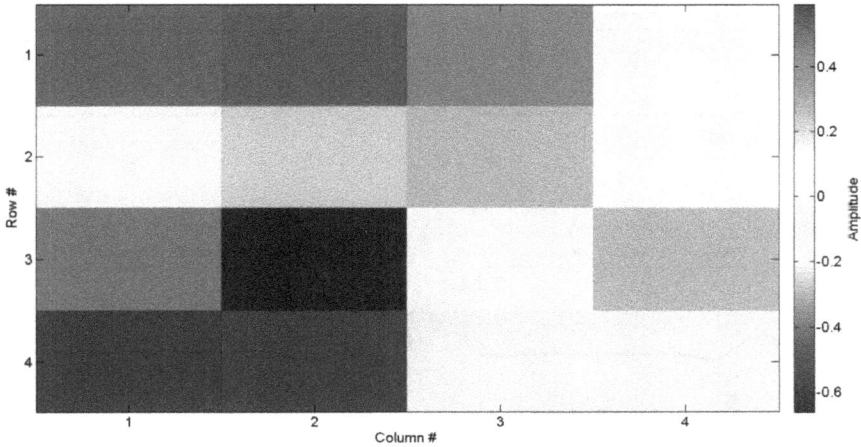

(a)

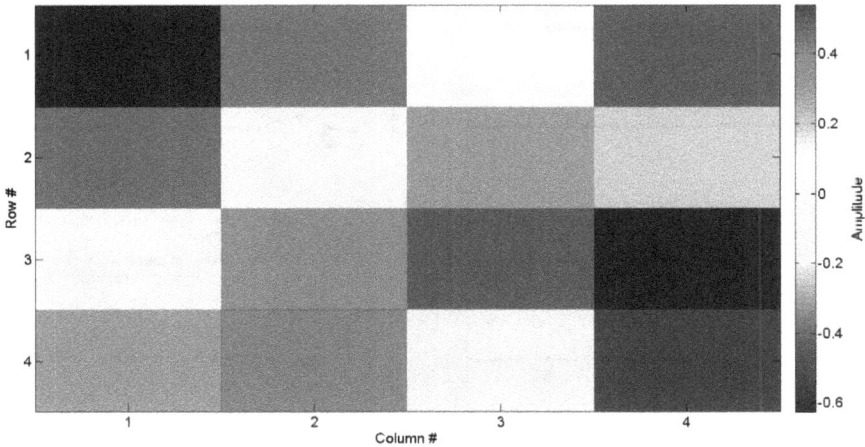

(b)

Figure 3.9 (a) Back-projection matrix [inverse of the unmixing matrix for extracting the independent components, as shown in Figure 3.4(a)]. (b) Back-projection matrix [inverse of the unmixing matrix for extracting the independent components, as shown in Figure 3.4(b)]. The unmixing matrices for producing the components shown in Figure 3.4 are under global optimization.

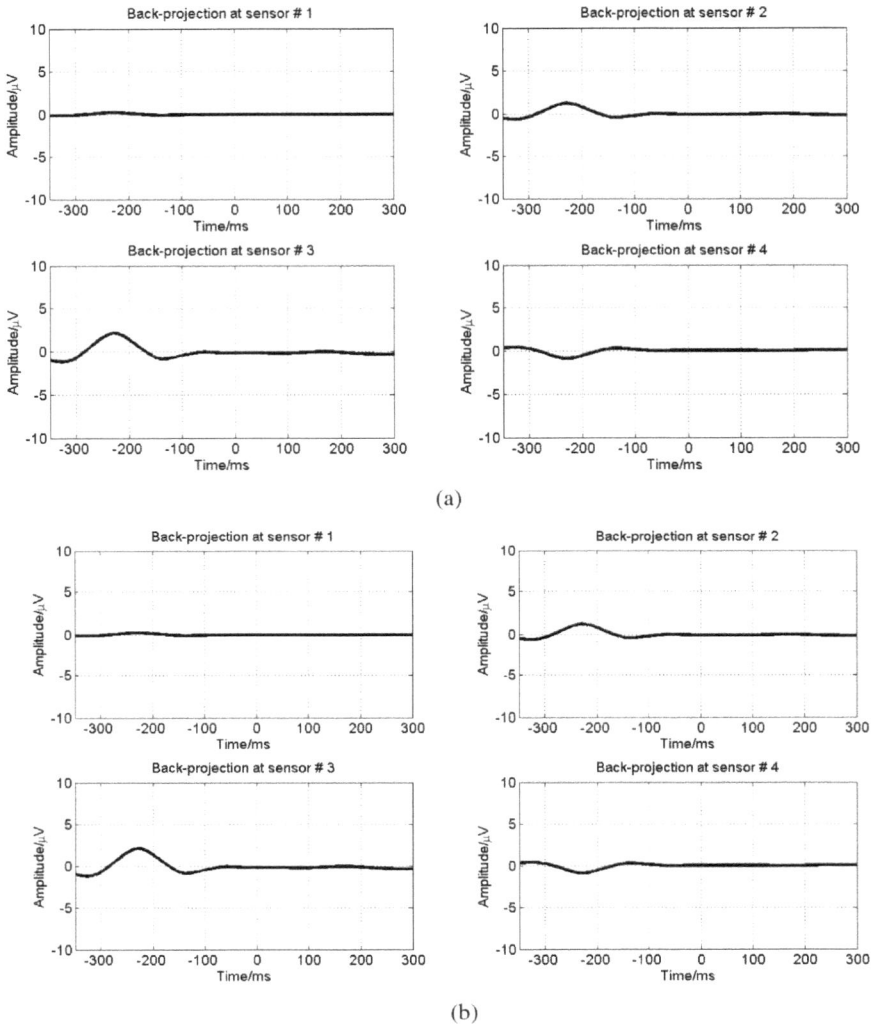

Figure 3.10 (a) Back-projection of component #4 shown in Figure 3.4(a). (b) Back-projection of component #3 shown in Figure 3.4(b). The unmixing matrices for producing the components shown in Figure 3.4 are under global optimization.

matrices are both under global optimization, and the two components are scaled versions of source #3 in Figure 3.2. Therefore, the back-projection of any of the two components is equal to the mapping of source# 3, as shown in Figure 3.5.

3.2.2.3 Back-projection under local optimization

In practice, it is very difficult for ICA to converge to the globally optimized points but it tends to converge to the locally optimized point. Therefore, we need to study the back-projection of an independent component under local optimization. In this case, more than one nonzero element exists in at least one row or one column of the global matrix. Equation (3-12) is then transformed into

$$y_q(t) = c_{q,\gamma_1} \cdot s_{\gamma_1}(t) + \cdots + c_{q,\gamma_p} \cdot s_{\gamma_p}(t) + \cdots + c_{q,\gamma_{P(q)}} \cdot s_{P(q)}(t)$$

$$= \sum_{p=1}^{P(q)} c_{q,\gamma_p} \cdot s_{\gamma_p}(t), \tag{3-25}$$

where $P(q)$ is the number of sources that exist in the qth independent component $y_q(t)$ and $P(q) \leq R$, $\gamma_p \in [1, R]$, $p = 1, \ldots, P(q)$.

After Eqs. (3-19) and (3-25) are substituted into Eq. (3-16), the back-projection of an independent component under local optimization is now expressed as

$$e_q(t) = b_q \cdot \sum_{p=1}^{P(q)} c_{q,\gamma_p} \cdot s_{\gamma_p}(t) \tag{3-26}$$

$$b_q = Ac_q \neq a_r c_{r,q}, \tag{3-27}$$

where a_r is the rth column of A ($r \to \forall[1, R]$) and c_q is the qth column of C.

Obviously, under local optimization, the back-projection of one independent component may still include more than one source, and it is still a mixture of more than one source and not a mapping of one source. Moreover, the topography of one independent component is not the scaled version of the mapping coefficients of a source. This fact means that a difference exists between the back-projection of one independent component and the mapping of one source.

The degree of difference depends on how well the mixtures are separated by the ICA. Quantitatively, it depends on the ratio of the maximal absolute value of any row/column of the global matrix and the second maximal absolute value of the row/column of the global matrix. The bigger the ratio is, the better is the separation by ICA, and the more the back-projection of one independent component is correlated with the mapping of one source (Cong, Kalyakin, & Ristaniemi, 2011; Cong, Kalyakin, Zheng, *et al.*, 2011).

Figure 3.11 shows the extracted independent components from the mixtures shown in Figure 3.2(b) when the ICA algorithm — here, FastICA (Hyvarinen, 1999) is used when the default parameters of the toolbox ICASSO (Himberg, Hyvarinen, & Esposito, 2004) — converges to the locally optimized points. Two examples of local optimization are shown. In contrast to the independent components extracted under global optimization shown in Figure 3.4, the independent components shown in Figure 3.11 are more or less still a mixture of a few sources. Figure 3.12 shows the similarity matrix among each set of the four independent components in Figure 3.11 and the four sources in Figure 3.2(a). In terms of the correlation coefficients in Figure 3.12, we can tell that the separation of the mixture shown in Figure 3.2(b) is satisfactory.

Figure 3.13 shows the global matrix and its inverse under local optimization. The global matrix is based on the mixing matrix shown in Figure 3.3(a) and the unmixing matrix for extracting the independent components shown in Figure 3.11(a). In each row and column, at least two nonzero elements are present, and Eq. (3-22) is no longer valid under local optimization. The independent component is still a mixture of some sources in terms of Eq. (3-25), and the (q, p) element of the global matrix is not the reciprocal of the (p, q) element of the inverse of the global matrix.

Figure 3.14 shows two back-projection matrices under local optimization. Equation (3-20) under global optimization is no longer valid under local optimization, which means that the column of the back-projection matrix under local optimization is not the scaled version of the column of the mixing matrix.

Figure 3.15 shows the back-projection of a selected independent component under local optimization and the mapping of the source that corresponds to the selected component. The back-projection and the mapping are no longer identical under local optimization. This condition is different from that under global optimization (shown in Figures 3.5 and 3.10).

Therefore, the back-projection of an independent component under local optimization is not 100% certain to correct the variance and polarity indeterminacies of the component.

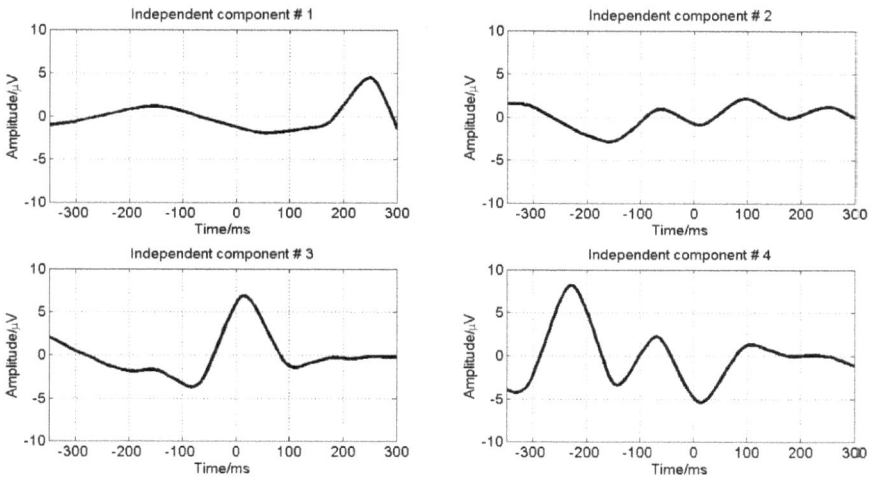

(a)

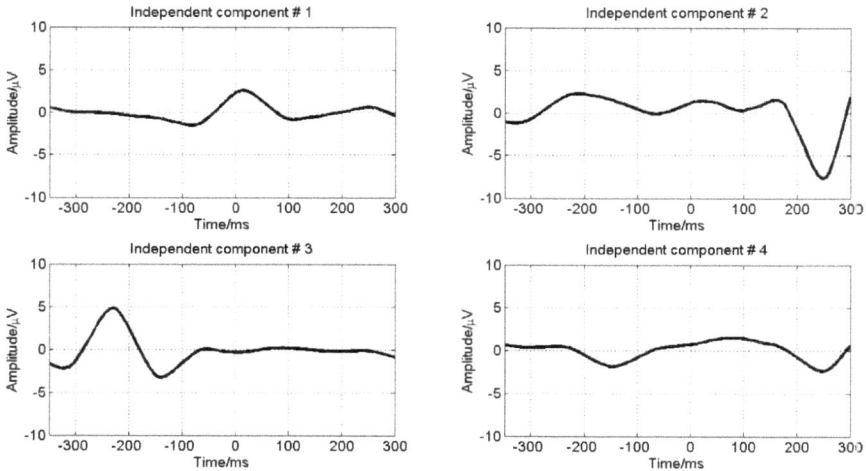

(b)

Figure 3.11 Extracted independent components when the ICA algorithm converges under local optimization. (a) and (b) Two cases with two different unmixing matrices and two different global matrices.

3.3 Indeterminacies and Determinacies of ICA on EEG

The variance and polarity of an independent component have been well known to be undetermined (Cichocki & Amari, 2003; Comon & Jutten,

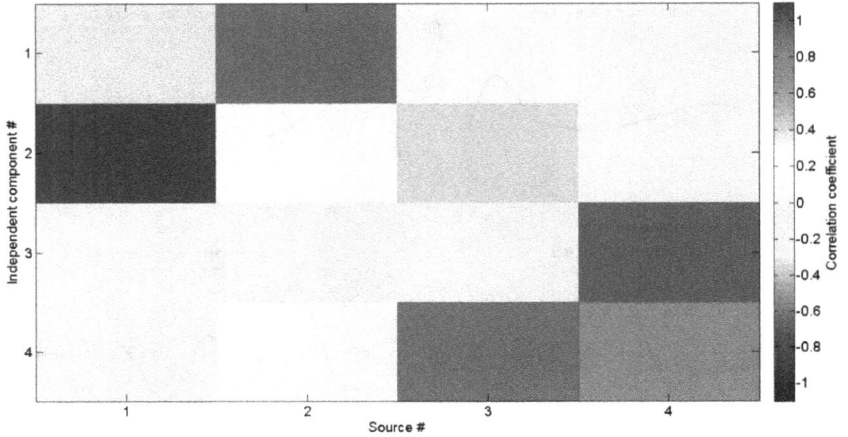

(a)

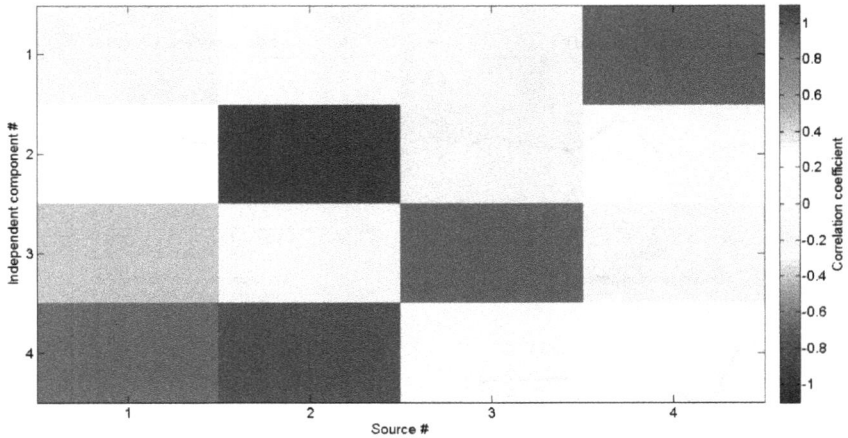

(b)

Figure 3.12   Similarity matrix between the extracted independent components and the sources. (a) Independent components shown in Figure 3.11(a). (b) Independent components shown in Figure 3.11(b). The sources are shown in Figure 3.2(a).

2010; Hyvarinen *et al.*, 2001). When ICA is applied to EEG data processing, the back-projection of the component has been generally acknowledged to possibly correct the indeterminacies (Makeig *et al.*, 1996, 1997; Makeig, Westerfield, Jung, *et al.*, 1999; Makeig, Westerfield, Townsend, *et al.*, 1999; Onton *et al.*, 2006).

(a)

(b)

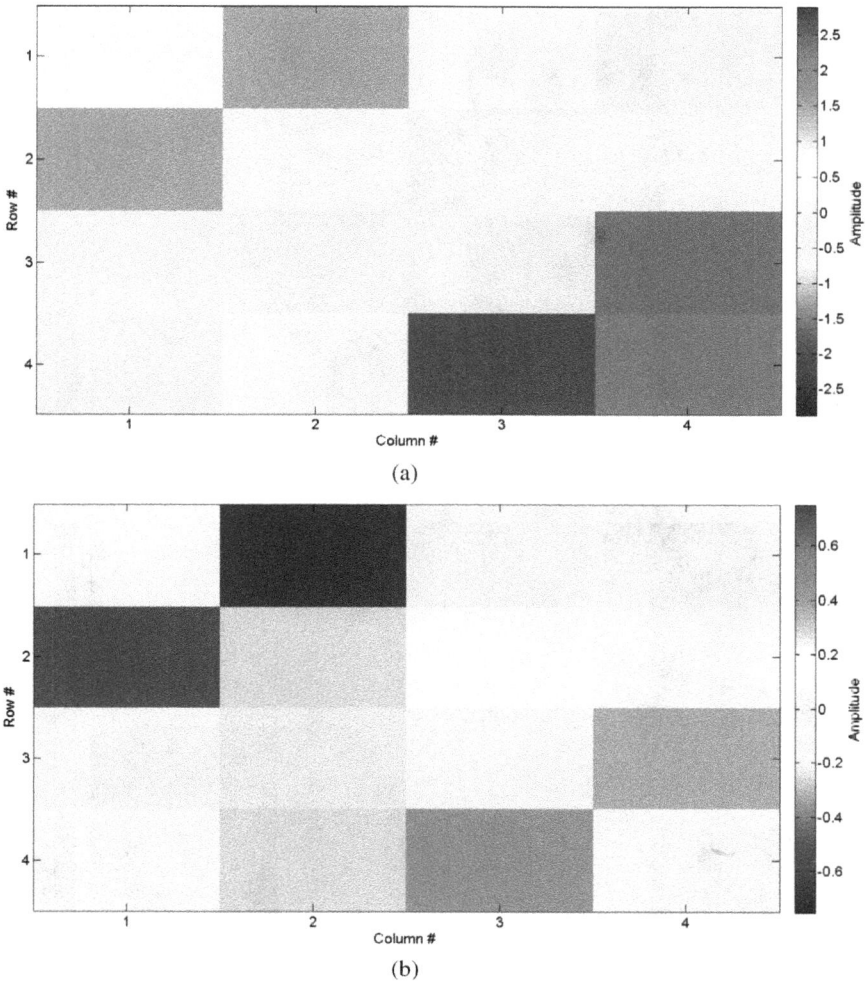

Figure 3.13 (a) Global matrix under local optimization. (b) Inverse of the global matrix in (a). The global matrix is based on the mixing matrix shown in Figure 3.3(a) and the unmixing matrix for extracting the independent components shown in Figure 3.11(a).

However, as we have discussed in Section 3.2, the back-projection cannot always succeed in correcting the indeterminacies.

Next, we summarize the indeterminacies and determinacies when ICA is applied to EEG data processing. In the discussion in the next section, we

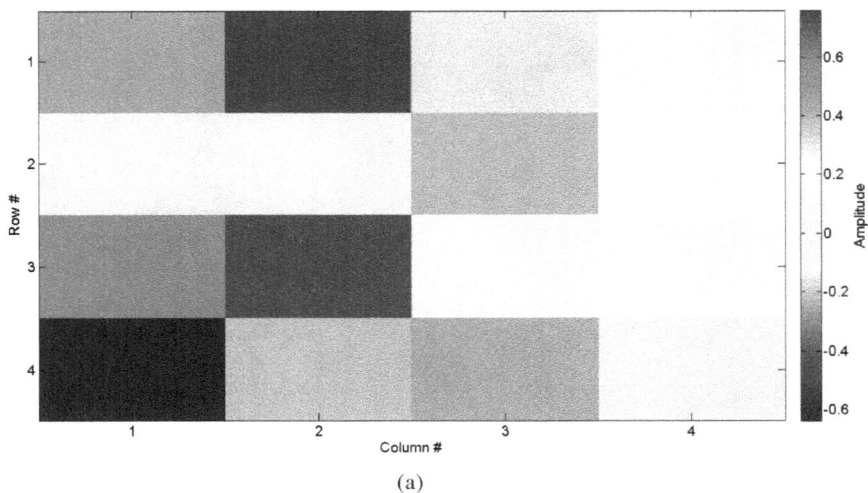

(a)

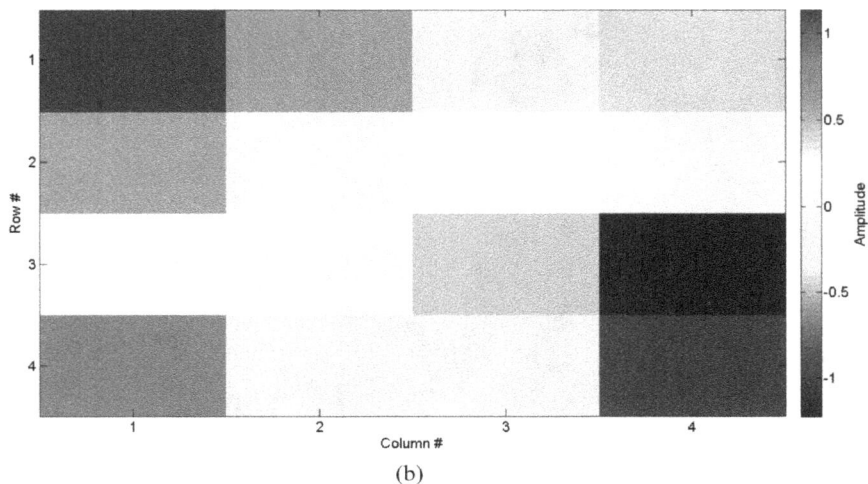

(b)

Figure 3.14   (a) Back-projection matrix [inverse of the unmixing matrix for extracting the independent components shown in Figure 3.11(a)]. (b) Back-projection matrix [inverse of the unmixing matrix for extracting the independent components shown in Figure 3.11(b)]. The unmixing matrices for generating the components shown in Figure 3.11 are under local optimization.

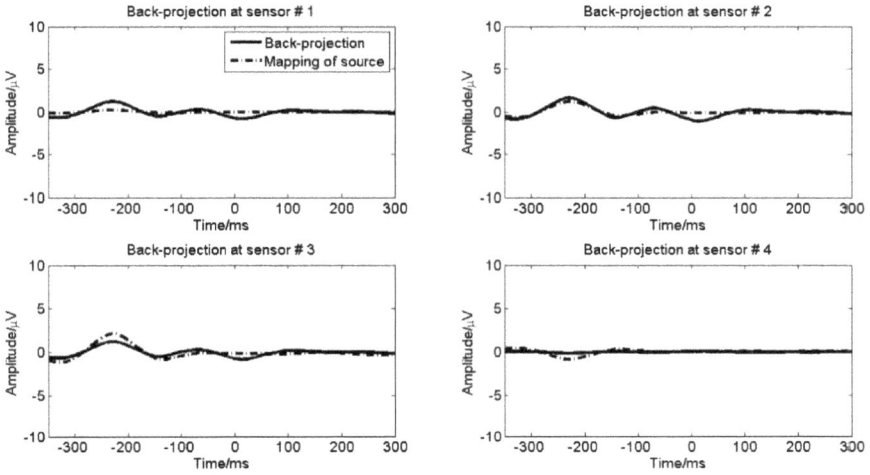

(a)

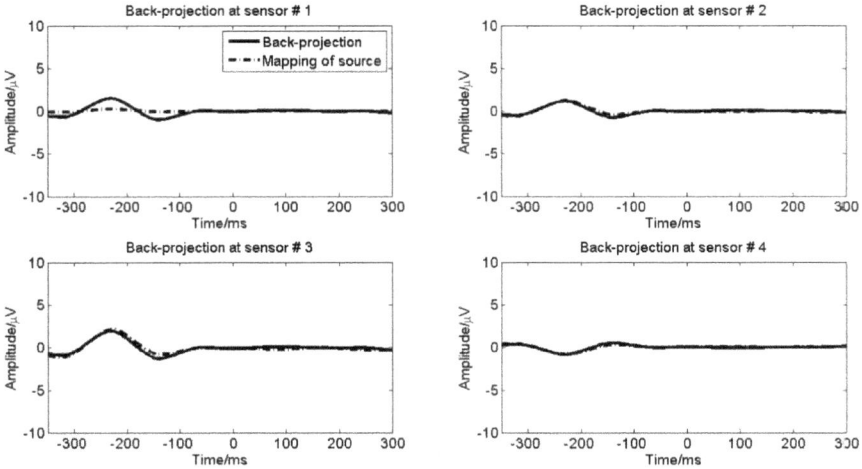

(b)

Figure 3.15 (a) Back-projection of component #4 in Figure 3.11(a). (b) Back-projection of component #3 in Figure 3.11(b). The unmixing matrices for generating the components shown in Figure 3.11 are under local optimization. The mapping of the source corresponding to the selected component is shown for comparison.

assume that an adaptive ICA algorithm with random initialization is applied to decompose the EEG data twice.

3.3.1 *Indeterminacies of ICA on EEG*

The indeterminacies result from two factors.

The first factor is related to the independent component. The orders of the components in two rounds may be different, and two selected components corresponding to the same source may have different variance and polarities, as shown in Figures 3.4 and 3.11. Such indeterminacies can appear under either the global or local optimization.

The other factor is related to the back-projection. With regard to the source of interest, the back-projection of a selected component in the first round may be different from that in the second round, and they are not identical to the mapping of the source, as shown in Figure 3.15. Such indeterminacies only occur under the local optimization.

3.3.2 *Determinacies in ICA on EEG*

The determinacies result from the back-projection under the global optimization.

In this optimization condition, the back-projection of a selected component in the first round is identical to that in the second round with regard to the source of interest, and they are the same as the mapping of the source. These determinacies are shown in Figure 3.10.

3.3.3 *Obtaining the determinacies of ICA on EEG in practice*

Obtaining the global optimization is not possible in practice. Thus, if obtaining the determinacies is difficult, applying ICA to the EEG/ERP data processing is inappropriate. However, we have learned that if the separation of the mixture by ICA into the source components is satisfactory, then obtaining quasi-determinacies is possible in practice.

In actual application, we do not know the true sources and the mixing matrix; thus, evaluating the extent of the separation by the ICA is not straightforward. In the following, we will introduce a systematic ICA approach to extract the ERP components from the ERP data of a subject under one condition and illustrate each step in detail.

3.4 Practical Consideration of the ICA Model of EEG

When ICA is applied on the EEG, we must take into account the EEG data properties. In the next section, we introduce two types of practical consideration for the ICA on the EEG.

3.4.1 *Noisy or noise-free ICA models*

In practice, sensor noise such as that expressed by Eq. (3-2) is always present. However, ICA algorithms are mostly designed for the noise-free model, thus creating a mismatch between the actual data and the employed ICA algorithms. Equation (3-1) can be converted into Eq. (3-2) to provide the rationale of using the noise-free ICA algorithms (Cong *et al.*, 2014).

Equation (3-1) can be written as follows:

$$
\begin{aligned}
z_m(t) &= a_{m,1} \cdot s_1(t) + \cdots + a_{m,R} \cdot s_R(t) + v_m(t) \\
&= a_{m,1} \cdot [s_1(t) + \boldsymbol{v}_{m,1}(t)] + \cdots + a_{m,R} \cdot [s_R(t) + \boldsymbol{v}_{m,R}(t)] \\
&= a_{m,1} \cdot \boldsymbol{s}_1(t) + \cdots + a_{m,R} \cdot \boldsymbol{s}_R(t),
\end{aligned}
\tag{3-28}
$$

$$
\boldsymbol{s}_r(t) = s_r(t) + \boldsymbol{v}_{m,r}(t),
\tag{3-29}
$$

$$
v_m(t) = a_{m,1} \cdot v_{m,1}(t) + \cdots + a_{m,r} \cdot \boldsymbol{v}_{m,r}(t) + \cdots + a_{m,R} \cdot \boldsymbol{v}_{m,R}(t)
\tag{3-30}
$$

Equation (3-28) indicates that in practice, the noisy sources $[\boldsymbol{s}_r(t), r = 1, 2, \ldots, R]$ can be extracted by ICA, expressing ICA in terms of the independence among the noisy sources $\boldsymbol{s}_r(t)[\boldsymbol{s}_r(t), r = 1, 2, \ldots, R]$. Indeed, noisy sources $\boldsymbol{s}_{r_1}(t)$ and $\boldsymbol{s}_{r_2}(t)$ can become dependent on each other provided that noise-free sources $s_{r_1}(t)$ and $s_{r_2}(t)$ are independent from each other. This condition may occur, particularly when the signal-to-noise ratio (SNR) is low.

Consequently, Eq. (3-28) implies that proper denoising can enhance the ICA decomposition.

3.4.2 *Can correcting artifacts and extracting the ERP components be realized simultaneously?*

ICA has been very successfully used to remove artifacts (Jung, Makeig, Humphries, *et al.*, 2000; Jung, Makeig, Westerfield, *et al.*, 2000; Lindsen & Bhattacharya, 2010; Mennes, Wouters, Vanrumste, Lagae, & Stiers, 2010; Vigario & Oja, 2008; Vigario, Sarela, Jousmaki, Hämäläinen, & Oja, 2000). For example, the open-source software EEGLAB (Delorme & Makeig, 2004) and commercial software such as Visional Analyzer (Brain Products GmbH) and BESA (BESA GmbH) have employed ICA to correct artifacts, including eye blinks and eye movements. Figure 3.16 shows one example (Jung, Makeig, Westerfield, *et al.*, 2000). After the ICA decomposition shown in Figure 3.7, two independent components are identified as artifact components. They are set to zero. After the back-projection, the artifacts are corrected.

ICA can also be used to extract the ERP components (Astikainen, Cong, Ristaniemi, & Hietanen, 2013; Bishop & Hardiman, 2010; Cong, Kalyakin, Li, *et al.*, 2011; Kalyakin, Gonzalez, Ivannikov, & Lyytinen, 2009; Kalyakin, Gonzalez, Kärkkäinen, & Lyytinen, 2008; Kovacevic & McIntosh, 2007; Lozano-Soldevilla, Marco-Pallares, Fuentemilla, & C., 2012; Makeig *et al.*, 1997; Marco-Pallares, Grau, & Ruffini, 2005; Vakorin, Kovacevic, & McIntosh, 2010; Vigario & Oja, 2008; Zeman,

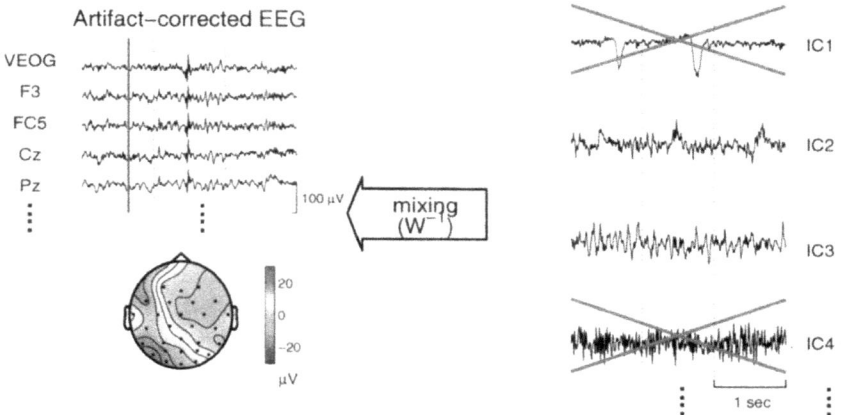

Figure 3.16 Example of using ICA for correcting artifacts on the basis of the ICA decomposition shown in Figure 3.7 [adapted from Jung, Makeig, Westerfield, *et al.* (2000)].

Till, Livingston, Tanaka, & Driessen, 2007). Therefore, a question arises on whether the ICA can simultaneously extract the artifacts and ERP components. The sources in the linear transform model in Eq. (3-1) include artifacts and ERP components. Theoretically, they can be simultaneously extracted by ICA. However, this extraction is hardly achieved in practice.

Artifacts, including eye movements and eye blinks, are usually much larger than the ERP sources. For example, the eye blink amplitudes can be over $100\,\mu$V, whereas the ERP amplitudes are usually smaller than $10\,\mu$V. When ICA is applied to correct artifacts, it is usually performed on continuous or concatenated single-trial EEG data, as shown in Figure 1.2. In these EEG data, the artifact source-to-noise ratio (SoNR) can be very high, but the ERP SoNR can be extremely low. According to Eq. (3-28), the noisy ERP sources may not be independent from each other in the continuous or concatenated single-trial EEG data, and the noisy artifact sources may still be independent from the noisy ERP sources. This condition indicates that the large artifact components can be successfully extracted, and the ERP components can hardly be extracted when ICA is applied to continuous or concatenated single-trial EEG data.

Therefore, simultaneously extracting the artifact and ERP components is very difficult. We suggest correcting or rejecting the artifacts first and then extracting the ERP components.

3.4.3 *Group- or individual-level ICA*

When ICA is applied to decompose EEG data, the EEG data of different subjects and under different conditions are often concatenated in the time domain (Delorme & Makeig, 2004) or stacked in the spatial domain (Eichele, Rachakonda, Brakedal, Eikeland, & Calhoun, 2011). In this manner, a group-level ICA is actually applied (Cong, He, *et al.*, 2013). The use of the group-level ICA features some advantages such as the following: (1) selecting the components of interest for different subjects is easier, (2) the data of different subjects are projected onto the same subspace, (3) the variance and polarity indeterminacies are not necessarily corrected, and (4) many samples for ICA decomposition are available.

Typically, everything has both an advantage and disadvantage. The group-level ICA requires additional assumptions (Cong, He, *et al.*, 2013).

Theoretically, the number of sources, the mixing matrices, and the order of sources of the different subjects should all be identical (Cong, He, *et al.*, 2013). These requirements limit the performance of the group-level ICA decomposition.

When ICA is employed on the EEG data of a single subject and under one condition, the application is called individual-level ICA, which means that no additional assumptions are made except those of the ICA theory (Section 3.1.2). The fewer the assumptions are, the more applicable is the signal processing approach. Moreover, for clinical application, performing signal processing on individual-level EEG data instead of group-level EEG data is very important. In the following, we introduce the method of using individual ICA to extract the ERP components from the ERP data (averaged EEG data over single trials) with a duration of one epoch/trial.

3.4.4 *Converting the over-determined model to the determined model*

Nowadays, the high-density EEG array that includes hundreds of electrodes is widely used for EEG data collection in ERP experiments. After the ERP data (averaged EEG over single trials) are obtained, we can reasonably assume that the number of sensors (e.g., electrodes) is larger than the number of sources in the data (Cong, He, Hämäläinen, Cichocki, & Ristaniemi, 2011; Cong, He, *et al.*, 2013). This means that the data model is over-determined. Then, we need to convert the over-determined model to the determined model before the ICA decomposition, as presented in Section 3.1.3. This process is called dimension reduction. The principal component analysis (PCA) (Jolliffe, 2002) can be applied for this purpose. PCA can be performed by eigenvalue decomposition of the sample covariance matrix of the data (Jolliffe, 2002).

Equation (3-3), namely, $\mathbf{x}(t) = \mathcal{A}\mathbf{s}(t)$, describes the over-determined model when $M > R$. Then, the sample covariance matrix of $\mathbf{x}(t)$ is given by

$$\Sigma = \frac{1}{T} \sum_{t=0}^{T-1} \mathbf{x}(t)\mathbf{x}^T(t), \tag{3-31}$$

where $\Sigma \in \Re^{M \times M}$ is a symmetric matrix and T is the number of samples.

To obtain the eigenvector and eigenvalue of the sample covariance matrix, an eigenvalue decomposition can be performed on Σ

$$\Sigma \Upsilon = \Lambda \Upsilon, \tag{3-32}$$

where $\Upsilon \in \Re^{M \times M}$ represents the M eigenvectors and each column of Υ is an eigenvector. Λ is a diagonal matrix, and each diagonal element denotes one eigenvalue. Moreover, the eigenvalues are ranked decreasingly.

Because only R sources are present, the first R eigenvectors compose the dimension-reduction matrix $\mathbf{V} \in \Re^{M \times R}$. Thus, the over-determined model can be converted to the determined model as follows:

$$\mathbf{x}(t) = \mathbf{V}^T \boldsymbol{\varkappa}(t) = \mathbf{V}^T \mathcal{A}\mathbf{s}(t) = \mathbf{A}\mathbf{s}(t) \tag{3-33}$$

$$\mathbf{V}^T \mathcal{A} = \mathbf{A}, \tag{3-34}$$

where $\mathbf{x}(t) = [x_1(t), x_2(t), \ldots, x_R(t)]^T \in \Re^{R \times 1}$ represents the virtual observation vector and denotes the first R principal components of $\boldsymbol{\varkappa}(t)$. $\mathbf{A} \in \Re^{R \times R}$ is a mixing matrix, which is a square matrix.

Therefore, determining the number of sources is very critical in practice to convert the over-determined model to the determined model. We will introduce solutions to this problem next.

3.4.5 *Converting the under-determined model to the determined model*

In the under-determined model, the number of sources is larger than the number of sensors. Therefore, to obtain the determined model, the number of sources should be reduced to the number of sensors, which is practically very difficult to achieve. We will illustrate this issue in this chapter.

3.5 MOS to Determine the Number of Sources

3.5.1 *Introduction to MOS*

Section 3.4.4 mentioned that precisely estimating the number of sources in the over-determined model is very critical for further ICA decomposition. Model order selection (MOS) can be applied for this estimation (Cong, He, *et al.*, 2011, 2013; Cong, Nandi, He, Cichocki, & Ristaniemi, 2012; Cong *et al.*, 2014).

MOS is an important and fundamental issue in a variety of signal processing applications (Abou-Elseoud *et al.*, 2010; Beckmann & Smith, 2004; Hansen & Yu, 2001; He, Cichocki, Xie, & Choi, 2010; Minka, 2001; Stoica & Selen, 2004). Generally, the MOS methods are derived from the information theory criteria (Akaike, 1974; Cavanaugh, 1999; Hansen & Yu, 2001; Liavas & Regalia, 2001; Liavas, Regalia, & Delmas, 1999; Rissanen, 1978; Stoica & Selen, 2004), Bayesian estimation (Minka, 2001; Schwarz, 1978; Seghouane & Cichocki, 2007), and on the basis of the gap in an ordered parameter sequence (Cong *et al.*, 2012; He *et al.*, 2010). The difficulties in MOS originate mainly from three factors, which include practical violation of the theoretical assumptions required by the method (Li, Adali, & Calhoun, 2007), short data (Kay, Nuttall, & Baggenstoss, 2001; Minka, 2001; Ulfarsson & Solo, 2008), and low SNR (Alkhaldi, Iskander, & Zoubir, 2010; He, Cichocki, & Xie, 2009; Selen & Larsson, 2007).

In the application of ICA on brain signals, the number of samples is usually large (Abou-Elseoud *et al.*, 2010; Cong, He, *et al.*, 2013; Cong *et al.*, 2014; Li *et al.*, 2007). However, the SNR of the brain signals is relatively low. In this chapter, we test the MOS on the basis of the simulated signals with SNR from -10 to 30 dB.

3.5.2 *Theoretical eigenvalues and MOS*

From Eqs. (3-1) and (3-3), the matrix-vector form of the ERP data model can be expressed as

$$\mathbf{z}(t) = \boldsymbol{\mathcal{A}}\mathbf{s}(t) + \boldsymbol{v}(t), \tag{3-35}$$

where $\mathbf{z}(t) = [z_1(t), z_2(t), \ldots, z_M(t)]^T \in \Re^{M \times 1}$ is the collected data vector by M sensors at one time stamp, $\boldsymbol{\mathcal{A}} \in \Re^{M \times R}$ is the mixing matrix, and $\mathbf{s}(t) = [s_1(t), s_2(t), \ldots, s_R(t)]^T \in \Re^{R \times 1}$ denotes the source vector.

We make the following three assumptions for MOS (He *et al.*, 2010): (1) $\boldsymbol{\mathcal{A}}$ is a tall matrix ($M > R$) and has a full column rank, i.e., the rank of $\boldsymbol{\mathcal{A}}$ is R; (2) noise signals $v_1(t), \ldots, v_M(t)$ are mutually independent and follow the identical Gaussian distribution $N(0, \sigma^2)$; and (3) the noise is statistically independent from the sources. Then, the theoretical covariance matrix is defined as

$$\boldsymbol{\Sigma}_{\mathbf{z}} = E[\mathbf{z}(t)\mathbf{z}(t)^T] = \boldsymbol{\mathcal{A}} \cdot \boldsymbol{\Sigma}_{\mathbf{s}} \cdot \boldsymbol{\mathcal{A}}^T + \sigma^2 \mathbf{I}, \tag{3-36}$$

where E denotes the *mathematical expectation*, $\mathbf{I}$ is the identity matrix, and $\mathbf{\Sigma_s} = E[\mathbf{s}(t)\mathbf{s}(t)^T]$. Because the rank of $\mathcal{A}$ is R, we can readily derive the following eigenvalue properties (He *et al.*, 2010; Liavas & Regalia, 2001; Liavas *et al.*, 1999; Wax & Kailath, 1985):

$$\lambda_{z,1} \geq \cdots \geq \lambda_{z,R} > \lambda_{z,R+1} = \cdots = \lambda_{z,M} = \sigma^2, \qquad (3\text{-}37)$$

where $\{\lambda_{z,m}\}_{m=1}^{M}$ are the eigenvalues of matrix $\mathbf{\Sigma_z}$ in the descending order.

Theoretically, because the last eigenvalue of covariance matrix $\mathbf{C_z}$ is duplicated $M - R$ times, we can straightforwardly obtain the number of sources in Eqs. (3-1) and (3-35).

In practice, we can obtain the sample covariance matrix defined by Eq. (3-31) but not the covariance matrix. We find that when the SNR is low, the smaller eigenvalues of $\mathbf{\Sigma_z}$ can be different, which results in failure to count the larger eigenvalues of the MOS. The selection of the number of components is sometimes based on the percentage of the explained variance by a certain number of eigenvalues over all eigenvalues, instead of using the MOS methods in terms of the linear transform model.

3.5.3 *MOS in practice*

Practically, the MOS for a linear transform model (He *et al.*, 2010) usually includes three steps: (1) calculating the eigenvalues of the sample covariance matrix, (2) computing the eigenspectrum on basis of the ordered eigenvalues, and (3) finding the minimum or maximum of the eigenspectrum to determine the number of sources. Therefore, the eigenspectrum derivation method is the key for the MOS. We next introduce the information-theory-criterion-based methods (Akaike, 1974; Cavanaugh, 1999; Rissanen, 1978). Second ORder sTatistic of the Eigenvalues (SORTE) (He *et al.*, 2010), and ratio of adjacent eigenvalues (RAE) (Cong *et al.*, 2012).

3.5.3.1 *Information-theory-based methods*

The Akaike's information criterion (AIC) (Akaike, 1974), minimum description length (MDL) (Rissanen, 1978), and Kullback–Leibler information criterion (KIC) (Cavanaugh, 1999) are used for comparison of the MOS. Indeed, AIC is the minimization of the Kullback–Leibler divergence between the true and fitted models, KIC uses the systematic

Kullback–Leibler divergence between the true and fitted models, and MDL is the minimum of the code length. They are defined as follows (Wax & Kailath, 1985):

$$E_{\text{AIC}}(m) = -2L(z|\Theta_m) + 2G(\Theta_m)$$

$$E_{\text{KIC}}(m) = -2L(z|\Theta_m) + 3G(\Theta_m)$$

$$E_{\text{MDL}}(m) = -L(z|\Theta_m) + \frac{1}{2}G(\Theta_m) \log \mathcal{T}$$

$$L(z|\Theta_m) = \frac{\mathcal{T}}{2} \log \left(\frac{\prod_{i=m+1}^{M} \lambda_{z,i}^{1/M-m}}{\frac{1}{M-m} \sum_{i=m+1}^{M} \lambda_{z,i}} \right)^{M-m}$$

$$G(\Theta_m) = 1 + Mm - \frac{1}{2}m(m-1),$$

where $\mathcal{T}$ is the number of samples, $L(z|\Theta_m)$ is the maximum log-likelihood of the observation on the basis of model parameter set Θ_m of the mth order, and $G(\Theta_m)$ is the penalty for the model complexity given by the total number of free parameters in Θ_m.

3.5.3.2 *SORTE*

To identify R by searching the gap between $\lambda_{z,R}$ and $\lambda_{z,R+1}$ in Eq. (3-37), a gap measure called SORTE is defined as follows (He *et al.*, 2010):

$$\text{SORTE}(m) = \begin{cases} \dfrac{var\left[\{\nabla\lambda_{z,i}\}_{i=m+1}^{M-1}\right]}{var\left[\{\nabla\lambda_{z,i}\}_{i=m}^{M-1}\right]}, & var\left[\{\nabla\lambda_{z,i}\}_{i=m}^{M-1}\right] \neq 0 \\ +\infty & var\left[\{\nabla\lambda_{z,i}\}_{i=m}^{M-1}\right] = 0 \end{cases},$$

where $m = 1, \ldots, (M-2)$.

$$var\left[\{\nabla\lambda_{z,i}\}_{i=m}^{M-1}\right] = \frac{1}{M-m} \sum_{i=m}^{M-1} \left(\nabla\lambda_{z,i} - \frac{1}{M-m}\sum_{i=m}^{M-1}\nabla\lambda_{z,i}\right)^2,$$

denotes the sample variance of the sequence $\{\nabla\lambda_{z,i}\}_{i=m}^{M-1}$, and $\nabla\lambda_{z,i} = \lambda_{z,i} - \lambda_{z,i+1}$, $i = 1, \ldots, (M-1)$. Then, we determine the number of sources using the following criterion: SORTE(R) is minimal (He *et al.*, 2010).

3.5.3.3 *RAE*

RAE was presented by Liavas and Regalia in 2001 (Liavas & Regalia, 2001). RAE appeared to have not been formally presented before. We have elaborated it in details (Cong *et al.*, 2012). RAE is expressed as

$$\text{RAE}(m) = \frac{\lambda_{z,m}}{\lambda_{z,m+1}}, m = 1, \ldots, (M-1).$$

Equivalently, we can define it as

$$\text{RAE}(m) = ln(\lambda_{z,m}) - ln(\lambda_{z,m+1}) = ln\frac{\lambda_{z,m}}{\lambda_{z,m+1}} \geq 0,$$

where $ln(\cdot)$ is the natural logarithm operation and $m = 1, \ldots, (M-1)$. By performing enough simulations, we can determine the number of sources using the following criterion: $\text{RAE}(R)$ is minimal when the SNR is high enough (Cong *et al.*, 2012).

Obviously, RAE is much more computationally efficient than SORTE, AIC, KIC, or MDL.

3.5.3.4 *Simulation for MOS*

In the simulations, the SNR is generally defined as

$$10\log_{10}\left(\sum_{m=1}^{M}\sum_{t=0}^{T-1} z(t)_m^2 \Big/ \sum_{m=1}^{M}\sum_{t=0}^{T-1} v(t)_m^2\right).$$

To express the relationship between the sources and the noise in the linear transform model, we define SoNR as

$$10\log_{10}\left[\left(\sum_{r=1}^{R}\sum_{t=0}^{T-1} s(t)_r^2 \Big/ R\right) \Big/ \left(\sum_{m=1}^{M}\sum_{t=0}^{T-1} v(t)_m^2 \Big/ M\right)\right].$$

The simulation procedure is shown by the pseudo MATLAB code in Figure 3.17 (Cong *et al.*, 2012).

Cong *et al.* (2012) stated that in the simulations, all sources in Eq. (3-1) with a unit variance had uniform distribution and were generated by the MATLAB command "rand". The noise in Eq. (3-1) had a Gaussian distribution and was generated by the MATLAB command "randn" and for the different sensors, the noise variance was kept identical. The noise

```
for n = 10:10:100 %% the number of sources
    for r = 5:10
        T = r*n²; %% number of samples
        for k =10:10:100
            m = n+k %% the number of sensors
            for SNR = -10:5:30 %% SNR
                x = As + e;
                Gain estimation for each method;
            end
        end
    end
end
```

Figure 3.17   Simulation procedure for the MOS (Cong *et al.*, 2012).

variance noise was determined by a predefined SNR. The mixing matrix in Eq. (3-1) was generated according to the MATLAB function "rand" and the mixing coefficients followed a uniform distribution between -1 and 1. Here, the relationship between the SoNR and SNR was not determined, but the SNR was definitely larger than the SoNR. The final results of the estimation of the number of sources were the average of 600 runs, including a loop of 10 runs for the number of sources, 6 runs for the number of samples, and 10 runs for the number of sensors, as shown in Figure 3.17.

For the RAE demonstrations, we first generated 10 sources and 30 observed signals through the model [Eq. (3-1)] with SoNR $= 4.7\,$dB and SNR $= 9.8\,$dB. Figure 3.18 shows the eigenvalues of the sample covariance matrices of the mixture, sample covariance matrix of the sources, variance in the noise, and eigenspectrum of the sample covariance matrix of the mixture, i.e., RAE. After maximizing the eigenspectrum, we found that the number of sources estimated by RAE was 10, which was the actual number of sources.

The example in Figure 3.18 shows that the SNR is high, and the signal at any sensor has larger energy than the corresponding noise. Three reasons are given for this. (1) The elements of the mixing matrix in this study conformed to the uniform distribution between -1 and 1. (2) The energy of the sources was invariant. (3) The energy of the noise among the different sensors was identical (Cong *et al.*, 2012).

Figure 3.19(a) shows the percentage error of the estimation when different MOS methods are used in the simulations. With regard to SORTE,

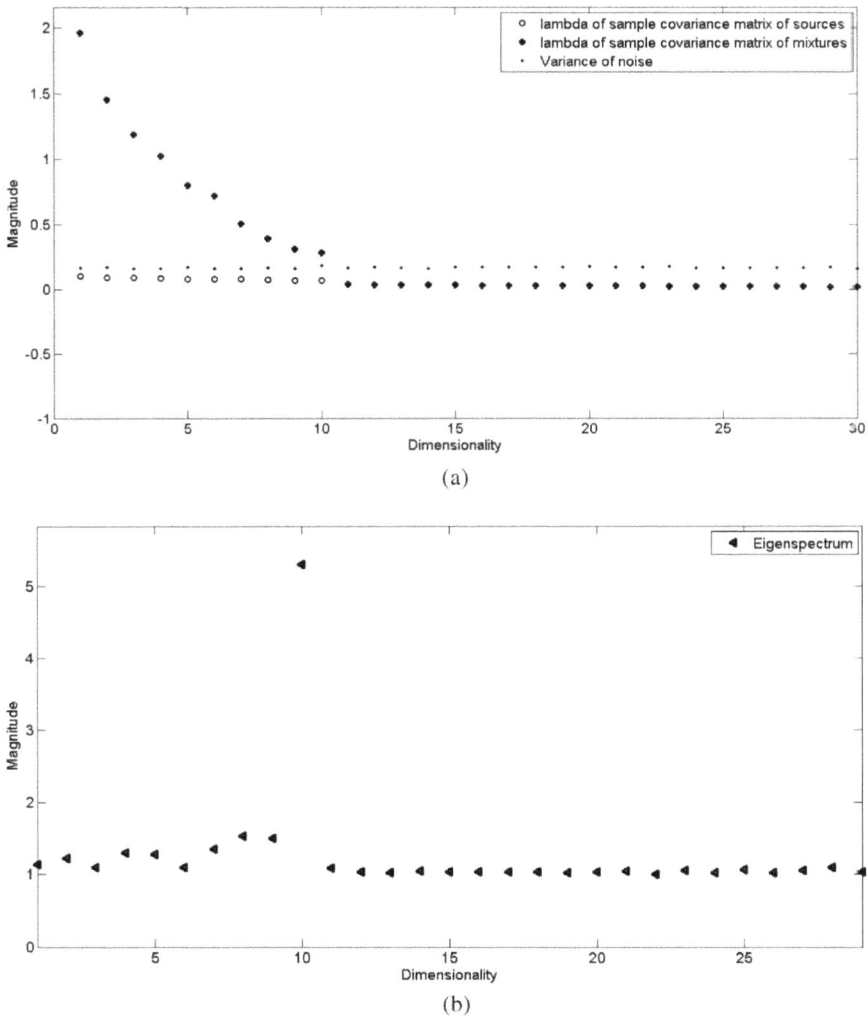

Figure 3.18   RAE demonstration. (a) Eigenvalues. (b) RAE eigenspectrum.

the error rate is more than 100% when the SNR is very low because the number of sensors in the simulation is much more than the number of sources, and the estimated number of sources is more than double the true number of sources. For the MDL and RAE, when the SNR is approximately $-10\,$dB, these methods indicate only a few sources in the noisy data.

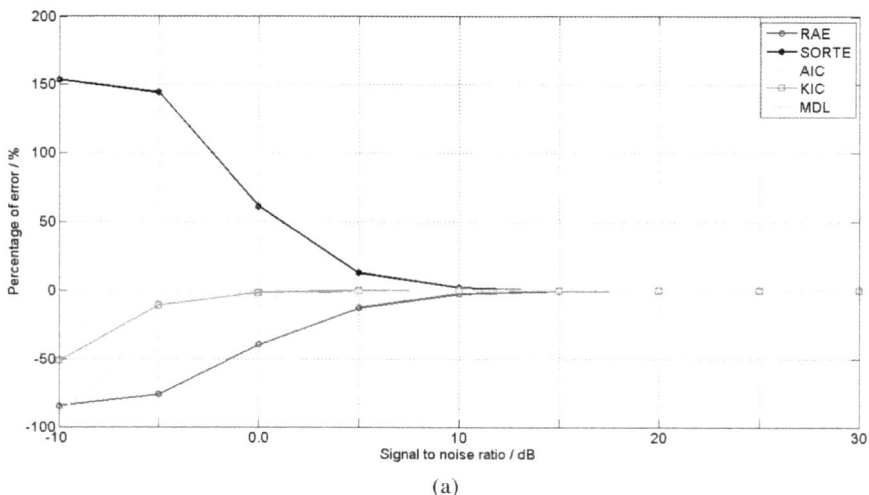

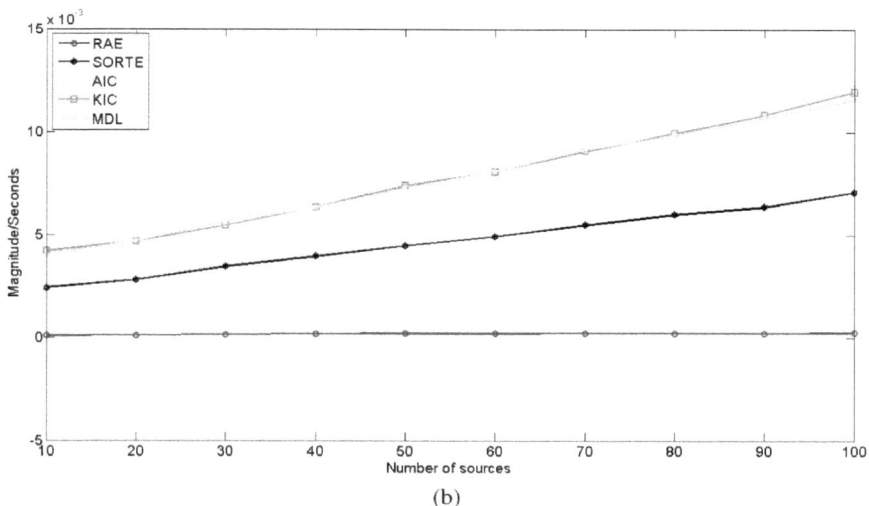

Figure 3.19   (a) Estimation of the MOS. (b) Time taken by the different methods.

Furthermore, Figure 3.19(b) shows that the time taken by SORTE is approximately half that required by AIC, KIC, and MDL. RAE is even more computationally efficient, and the time taken by RAE is almost negligible in contrast to the other methods. Hence, RAE is computationally efficient, which is very useful in real-time signal processing (Cong *et al.*, 2012).

In the simulations, the energy of the different sources is kept identical, and the energy of the noise of the different sensors remains invariable, which is convenient for the SNR calculation. In practice, the energy of the different sources can be different, and the energy of the noise of the different sensors in different locations can vary. Furthermore, the noise distribution may not be white Gaussian, and some sources might be correlated with one another, e.g., the EEG data recorded along the scalp and the acoustic data recorded by a microphone array. Hence, to investigate the MOS in order to determine the number of sources for a specific problem, we need to properly design the simulation for practical application (Cong *et al.*, 2012).

The simulation study also indicates that the MOS can be very accurate when the SNR is sufficiently high. Therefore, in practice, denoising the collected data before the MOS is very necessary for precise estimation.

3.6 Key Practical Issues for ICA to Extract the ERP Components

3.6.1 *Are the concatenated single-trial or averaged EEG data better for ICA to extract the ERP components under the assumption of independence?*

Figure 1.2 shows the existence of four EEG data types. They are the continuous EEG data, concatenated single-trial EEG data, EEG data of one single trial, and averaged EEG data over single trials in ERP experiments. Initial ICA application on the EEG data is performed on the averaged EEG data (Makeig *et al.*, 1996, 1997). When EEGLAB was developed, ICA has been increasingly applied on concatenated single-trial EEG data (Delorme & Makeig, 2004). Recently, some studies have applied ICA on the EEG data of one single trial (Cong *et al.*, 2010; Iyer & Zouridakis, 2007) and averaged EEG data over single trials (Cong, Kalyakin, Li, *et al.*, 2011; Kalyakin *et al.*, 2008, 2009).

After the ICA is performed on the concatenated single-trial EEG data, one ICA component is disconnected into single trials, and the EEG data in the component space are then averaged over single trials (Delorme & Makeig, 2004). In reality, the application of ICA on the concatenated single-trial EEG data is classified as a group-level ICA (Cong, He, *et al.*, 2013). Theoretically, no difference exists between the application of ICA on the concatenated single-trial EEG data and averaging the single trials in the component space and that on the averaged EEG data over single trials (Cong & Ristaniemi, 2011). The SNR of the single-trial EEG data tends to be much lower than that in the averaged EEG data. According to Eq. (3-28), the sources to be extracted by ICA are the noisy sources. Obviously, the extent of independence among the noisy sources in Eq. (3-28) is severely weakened in contrast to that among the noise-free sources in Eq. (3-1). Therefore, from the viewpoint of satisfying the ICA assumptions, applying the ICA on the averaged EEG data instead of the concatenated single-trial EEG data is more plausible.

3.6.2 *Number of samples and number of sources*

Practically, a limitation exists between the number of samples and the number of sources extracted by ICA. The former should be at least several times the square of the latter when ICA is applied on the averaged EEG (Makeig *et al.*, 1996, 1997; Makeig, Westerfield, Jung, *et al.*, 1999; Makeig, Westerfield, Townsend, *et al.*, 1999). On the other hand, the former should be at least 20 times the square of the latter when ICA is applied on the concatenated single-trial EEG data (Onton *et al.*, 2006).

In ERP experiments, the duration of the averaged EEG over single trials is only one epoch and is usually less than 1 s. The sampling frequency in ERP experiments is usually 1000, 500, or 250 Hz. Then, the number of samples in each epoch tends to be less than 1000. As a result, if ICA is applied on the averaged EEG, the ICA should extract only a few dozens of sources.

3.6.3 *Reducing the number of sources in averaged EEG data and increasing the SNR*

3.6.3.1 *Filtering the averaged EEG data*

The averaged EEG data can be modeled by Eq. (3-1). When a linear filter (e.g., a digital or wavelet filter) is applied on the averaged EEG, the output can be modeled in terms of Eqs. (3-1) and (3-28) as

$$\tilde{z}_m(t) = f[z_m(t)]$$
$$= f[a_{m,1} \cdot s_1(t) + \cdots + a_{m,r} \cdot s_r(t) + \cdots + a_{m,R} \cdot s_R(t) + v_m(t)]$$

$$= f[a_{m,1} \cdot s_1(t)] + \cdots + f[a_{m,R} \cdot s_R(t)] + f[\upsilon_m(t)]$$
$$= a_{m,1} \cdot f[s_1(t)] + \cdots + a_{m,R} \cdot f[s_R(t)] + f[\upsilon_m(t)]$$
$$= a_{m,\gamma_1} \cdot \mathbf{s}_{\gamma_1}(t) + \cdots + a_{m,\gamma_p} \cdot \mathbf{s}_{\gamma_p}(t) + \cdots + a_{m,\gamma_P} \cdot \mathbf{s}_P(t)$$

$$\mathbf{s}_{\gamma_p}(t) = f[s_{\gamma_p}(t)] + f[\mathbf{v}_{m,\gamma_p}(t)]$$

$$f[\upsilon_m(t)] = a_{m,\gamma_1} \cdot f[\mathbf{v}_{m,\gamma_1}(t)] + \cdots + a_{m,\gamma_P} \cdot f[\mathbf{v}_{m,\gamma_P}(t)], \qquad (3\text{-}38)$$

where P is the number of sources that still exists in the filtered averaged EEG data and $P \le R$. $\gamma_1 < \gamma_2 < \cdots < \gamma_p < \cdots < \gamma_P$, $p = 1, \ldots, P$, and $\gamma_p \in [1, R]$.

Equation (3-38) indicates four points.

(1) The linear filter does not change the coefficient between the source and the point along the scalp.
(2) The linear filter can remove some sources whose frequency components are outside the pass band of the filter.
(3) The linear filter can remove parts of some sources whose partial frequency components are outside the pass band of the filter.
(4) The linear filter can remove parts of the additive noise.

Consequently, the number of sources in appropriately filtered averaged EEG data may become smaller than that before the filtering. Furthermore, the SNR in the data can be improved. These are the benefits of the application of an appropriate filter on the averaged EEG data.

3.6.3.2 *Appropriately designed wavelet filter*

Designing an appropriate filter is thus very important, as expressed by Eq. (3.38). The ERP properties should be considered in the filter design.

ERPs have been acknowledged to have very low frequency components, and its main power falls below 10 Hz (Kalyakin *et al.*, 2007; Rossion & Jacques, 2008). However, this fact does not mean that the power of ERPs above 10 Hz is not important. In ERP experiments, spontaneous brain activity can also occur simultaneously, in addition to the brain activity elicited by the stimuli. Therefore, spontaneous EEG and ERPs overlap in the frequency domain. As introduced in Chapter 2, a digital filter cannot separate the overlapped frequency components of the two signals, but a wavelet filter can possibly achieve this process.

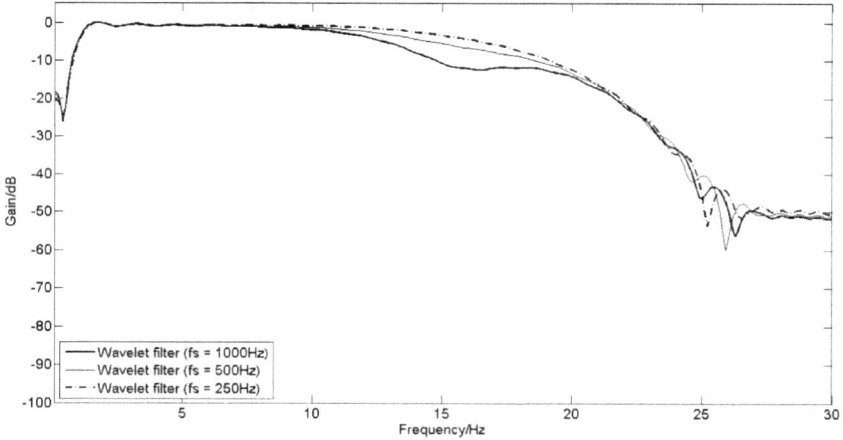

(a)

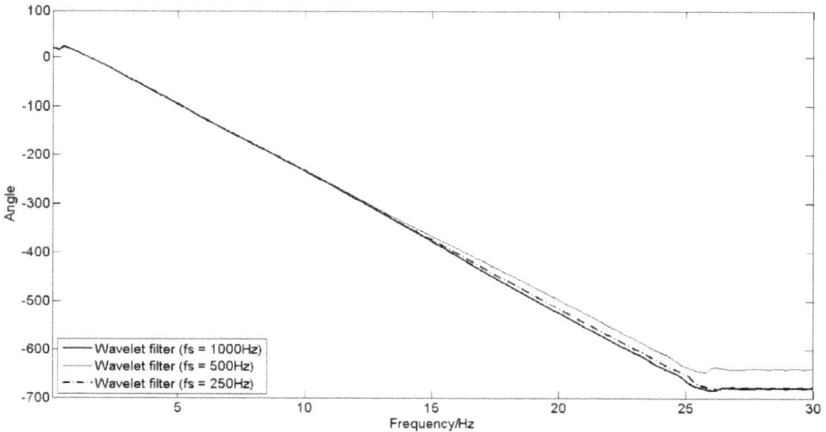

(b)

Figure 3.20 Three appropriate wavelet filters: (a) Magnitude responses. (b) Phase responses. For sampling frequencies of 1000, 500, and 250 Hz, the numbers of levels of the wavelet filters are 10, 9 and 8, and the level numbers for the wavelet filters are [9, 8, 7 ,6], [8, 7, 6, 5], and [7, 6, 5, 4], respectively. The wavelet for the filter is reverse biorthogonal 6.8 (rbio6.8).

Figure 3.20 shows examples of three appropriate wavelet filters under three sampling frequencies. The appropriate wavelet filters remove the very low frequency components (less than 0.5 Hz) and the very high frequency components (higher than 25 Hz) of the averaged EEG data. From 0.5 to

1.5 Hz and from 10 to over 20 Hz, some of the low-frequency drifts and higher frequency oscillations are partially removed from the ordinarily averaged EEG data. For example, the alpha and beta oscillations are partially removed. Meanwhile, the noise is also reduced.

3.6.4 *Validation of the stability of ICA decomposition*

Most ICA algorithms are adaptive. For example, one adaptive algorithm converges after a predefined threshold of some criterion is met, as introduced in Section 3.1.3.3 (implementation of the ICA algorithm). In fact, different mixing matrices can satisfy the criterion, as shown in Figure 3.4. For example, if an adaptive ICA algorithm is applied on the same dataset twice, we must know if the two sets of ICA components are similar or not.

Figure 3.21 shows the similarity matrix between the independent components of the two sets shown in Figure 3.4. Because the independent components are highly correlated with each other, we know that the ICA decomposition is stable. However, in high-dimensional space, the similarity matrix is not an ideal solution to examine the stability of multiple runs of ICA decomposition. Instead, clustering (Bishop, 2006) is applied in the examination (Groppe, Makeig, & Kutas, 2009; Himberg *et al.*, 2004; Hyvarinen, 2011, 2013; Hyvarinen & Ramkumar, 2013).

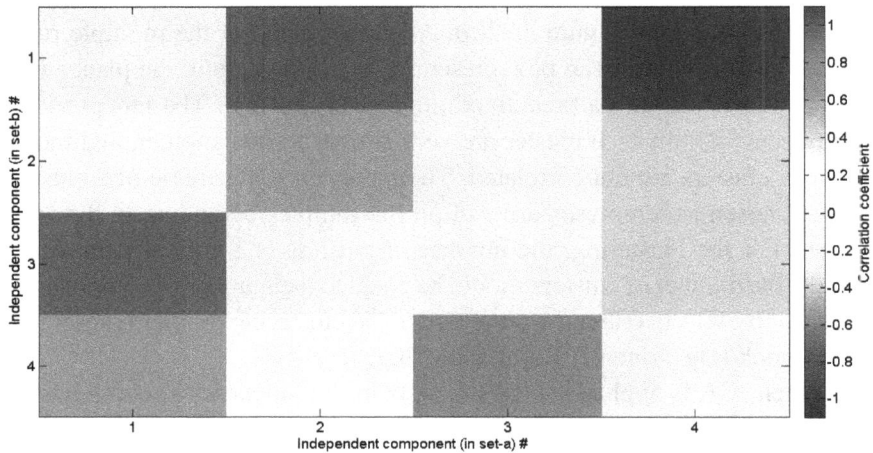

Figure 3.21   Similarity matrix between the independent components of two sets.

(a) Original points   (b) Two clusters.

(c) Four clusters.   (d) Six clusters.

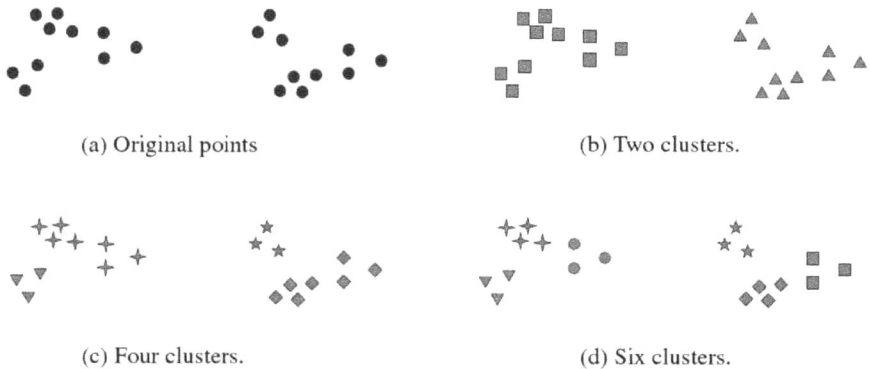

Figure 3.22   Examples of clustering (Tan, Steinbach, & Kumar, 2005). Each dot in (a) represents one data sample for clustering. In this book, each dot denotes one independent component.

Figure 3.22 shows a clustering example (Tan, Steinbach, & Kumar, 2005). For instance, all dots in Figure 3.22(a) can be clustered into a predefined number of clusters, e.g., two, as shown in Figure 3.22(b). If the clustering is performed well, the samples within each cluster are similar, and the samples between the clusters are different. Figures 3.22(b)–(d) show the results where all samples are clustered into different numbers of clusters.

We can adapt the example shown in Figure 3.22 to the problem presented in this book. In this example, one independent component is represented by one dot, as shown in Figure 3.22(a). All components of the multiple runs of ICA decomposition can be represented by all the dots in the plane, and they are clustered into a predefined number of clusters. The independent components within each cluster are very similar to one another, and those between clusters are not correlated. Then, the centroid sample of a cluster can be chosen as a representative of all the samples belonging to the said cluster. For the clustering, the number of clusters is a critical parameter. Ideally, the number of clusters should be equal to the number of components extracted by ICA in one run with regard to the clustering problem presented in this book (Hyvarinen & Ramkumar, 2013).

When ICA is applied on the ERPs, both the independent components and the corresponding topographies are important. Currently, the stability of the ICA decomposition is usually examined by the clustering results of the independent components (Himberg *et al.*, 2004).

3.7 Systematic ICA Approach on the Extraction of ERP Components from Averaged EEG Data (Responses of Stimuli) Collected by a High-Density Array

In this section, we will show how ICA can be used to extract the ERP components from the averaged EEG data of one subject and under one condition. The duration of the ERP data is one epoch, and the ERP data are collected by a high-density array. The ERP data used here are elicited by a passive oddball paradigm, which includes one type of standard stimuli and two types of deviant stimuli in the ratio 90/10/10. The standard stimulus is /ba/, and the two deviant stimuli are /ga/ and /da/ (Landi, 2012). This paradigm is used to elicit mismatch negativity (MMN). The deviant (/ga/) responses of a healthy child are used as an example. The child is approximately 10 years old. In the following, we illustrate the six steps of the systematic ICA approach.

3.7.1 *Ordinary ERP data: Ordinarily averaged EEG data over single trials of one stimulus and one subject*

The data were collected by the Electrical Geodesics Inc. netAmps 3 system using 128-Ag–AgC1-electrode nets and employing a sampling rate of 500 Hz. Each epoch started 100 ms before the stimulus onset and stopped 600 ms after the stimulus onset. After the conventional filtering (0.01–30 Hz), the EEG data were segmented into epochs. Next, artifact detection and rejection were performed on the segmented EEG data. For each epoch, the EEG data of those channels with minimum and maximum amplitudes exceeding $200 \mu V$ during the epoch (either due to eye blinks, eye movements, or movement artifact) were replaced using spherical spline interpolation on the basis of the data of the other channels. When the number of channels is greater than 10% of the channels required for the interpolation, the whole EEG epoch was excluded. Finally, the data were run through baseline correction and averaging before being exported and loaded into MATLAB for further analysis. For the data collection, Cz was used as the reference electrode.

Figure 3.23(a) shows the ERP waveforms under the conventional data processing (ordinary averaging), wavelet filtering, and systematic ICA approach. The solid curve represents the ordinarily averaged EEG data,

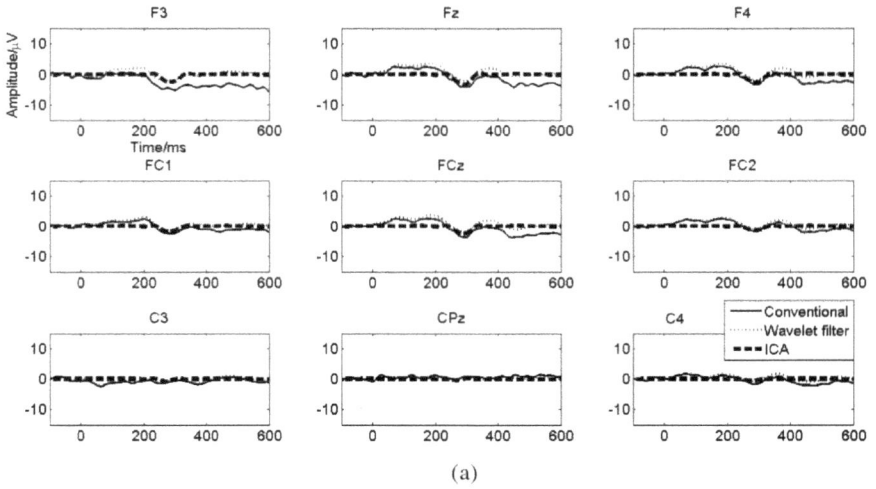

(a)

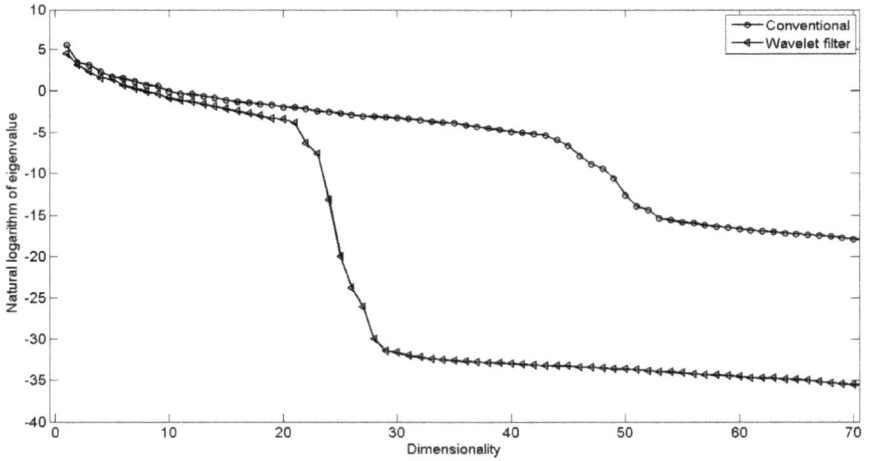

(b)

Figure 3.23 (a) ERP waveforms. (b) Natural logarithm of the eigenvalues. In (a), "Conventional" means the ordinarily averaged EEG data, i.e., ERP data; "Wavelet filter" means the wavelet-filtered ERP data; and "ICA" means the spatially filtered ERP data by the systematic ICA approach.

i.e., ERP data. The waveforms are sufficient because they are averaged over approximately 100 single trials and are deviant responses.

3.7.2 *Wavelet filtering of averaged EEG data*

The dotted curve in Figure 3.23(a) represents the wavelet-filtered averaged EEG data. The wavelet filter is the one shown in Figure 3.20 when the sampling frequency is 500 Hz. Figure 3.23(b) shows the natural logarithms of the eigenvalues of the sample covariance matrix of the ordinarily averaged EEG data and those of the sample covariance matrix of the wavelet-filtered averaged EEG data. Figure 3.23(b) shows the eigenspectra of the MOS method, which are the RAE presented in Section 3.5.3.3, to determine the number of sources in the data. For clarity of the plots, only the first 70 of the 128 eigenvalues are shown.

The breaking points of the eigenvalues of the wavelet-filtered averaged EEG data and the ordinarily averaged EEG data respectively appear on eigenvalues #20−#30 and eigenvalues #40−#50. Therefore, in terms of the frequency response of the wavelet filter, we can conclude that the wavelet filter has removed some uninteresting sources. We should note that the baseline of the wavelet-filtered averaged EEG data is removed after the ordinarily averaged EEG data are filtered. This is the normal preprocessing step before the ERP amplitude is measured and is intended for fair comparison among the different methods.

3.7.3 *Converting the over-determined model to the determined model: Dimension reduction*

Using RAE, we estimate that 21 sources exist in the wavelet-filtered averaged EEG data. Then, the over-determined linear transform model is converted into the determined model using Eqs. (3-31)–(3-33). Figure 3.24(a) shows the first 21 principal components of the wavelet-filtered averaged EEG data. The 21 principal components are the 21 virtual channel data, which conform to the determined linear transform model. These 21 principal components are the mixture that the ICA will separate.

To demonstrate the benefit of the wavelet filter proposed in this book, Figure 3.24(b) shows the 21 principal components of the ordinarily averaged

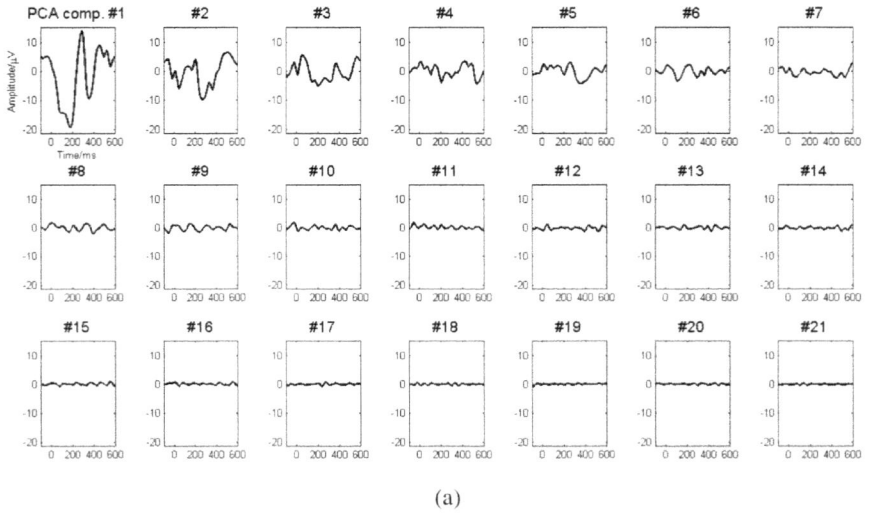

(a)

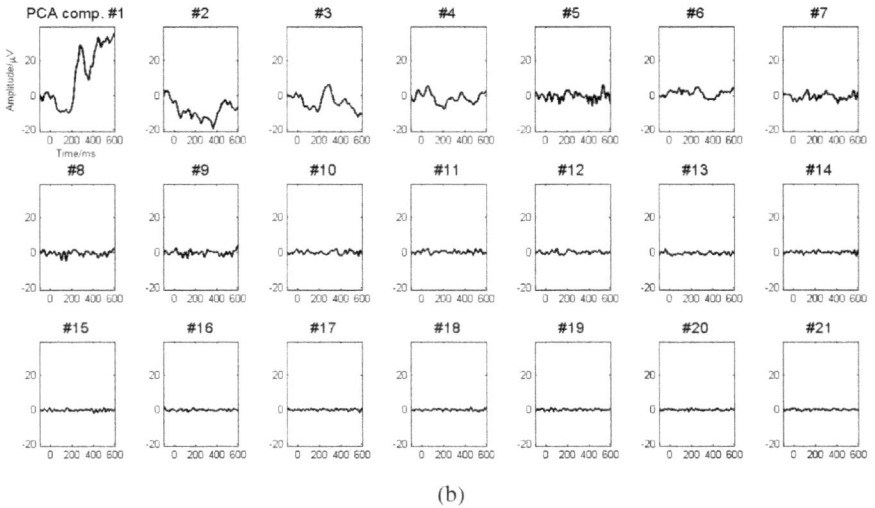

(b)

Figure 3.24   (a) 21 PCA components of the wavelet-filtered averaged EEG data. (b) 21 PCA components of the ordinarily averaged EEG data.

EEG data. They are noisier than the first 21 principal components of the wavelet-filtered averaged EEG data.

3.7.4 *ICA decomposition and stability analysis*

For the ICA decomposition in Eq. (3-7), the FastICA-based (Hyvarinen, 1999) ICASSO software (Himberg *et al.*, 2004) is used in this study. Using ICASSO, the FastICA is run 100 times using a randomly initialized unmixing matrix for each run, and all extracted independent components of the 100 runs are clustered. We use the "*tanh*" nonlinear function of the FastICA. The number of sources is 21, and the number of clusters is 21. For the other ICASSO and FastICA parameters, the default values are used. After the clustering, the independent component at the centroid of the cluster is selected as a representative component of the cluster. After the independent components are generated, their topographies can be obtained as

$$\mathbf{T} = \mathbf{VB} = \mathbf{VW}^{-1}, \tag{3-39}$$

where $\mathbf{T} \in \mathfrak{R}^{M \times R}$ and each column carries the independent component topography.

Figure 3.25 shows the 21 independent components extracted by the ICA from the 21 PCA components of the wavelet-filtered averaged EEG data and their corresponding topographies. The components are ordered according to the increasing peak latencies. From the BSS viewpoint, the sources are very well separated because the extracted independent components represent a sole peak. Most topographies show a dipolar brain activity, indicating that the ICA decomposition is very reliable (Delorme, Palmer, Onton, Oostenveld, & Makeig, 2012). For comparison, ICA decomposition is performed on the 21 principal components of the ordinarily averaged EEG data. Figure 3.26 shows the 21 independent components and their topographies. In contrast to the 21 independent components from the wavelet-filtered averaged EEG data, those from the ordinarily averaged EEG data are much noisier, indicating that the analysis using Eq. (3-28) in Section 3.4.1 is reasonable. Furthermore, the topographies of the 21 independent components from the ordinarily averaged EEG data are more scattered than those from the wavelet-filtered averaged EEG data, indicating

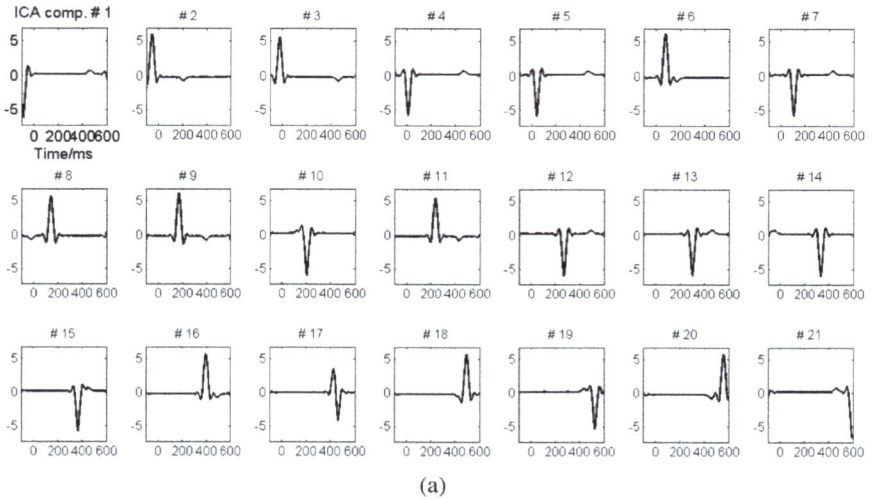

(a)

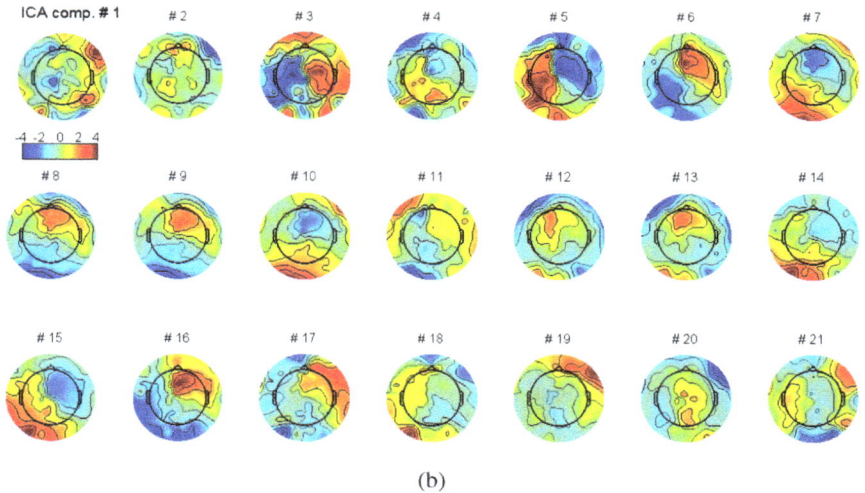

(b)

Figure 3.25 (a) 21 independent components extracted by the ICA from the 21 PCA components of the wavelet-filtered averaged EEG data. (b) 21 topographies of the 21 independent components extracted by the ICA from the 21 PCA components of the wavelet-filtered averaged EEG data. The variance and polarity of any component or topography are not determined in (a) and (b). The components are ordered according to their latencies.

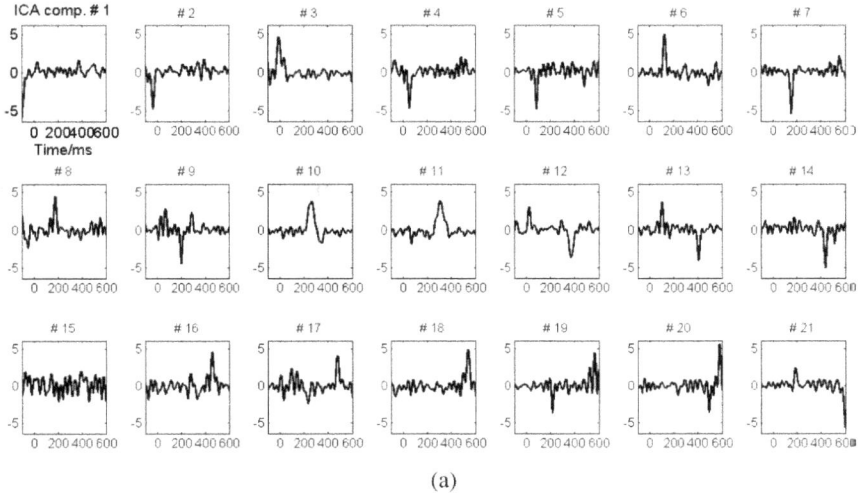

(a)

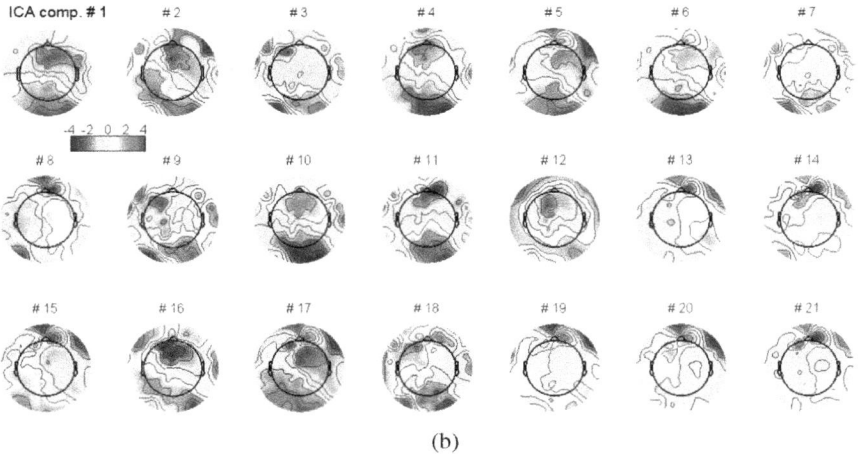

(b)

Figure 3.26 (a) 21 independent components extracted by the ICA from the 21 PCA components of the ordinarily averaged EEG data. (b) 21 topographies of the 21 independent components extracted by the ICA from the 21 PCA components of the ordinarily averaged EEG data. The variance and polarity of any component or topography are not determined in (a) and (b). The components are ordered according to their latencies.

that the findings from the averaged EEG data are less reliable. This is because reliable independent components should correspond to the locally focused topography resulting from dipolar brain activity (Delorme *et al.*, 2012).

We should note that the sampling frequency of the principal components is increased four times to increase the number of samples in the ICA decomposition. After the independent components are extracted, they are downsampled to the original sampling frequency.

Furthermore, the stability analyses of the independent components in Figures 3.25 and 3.26 are shown in Figures 3.27 and 3.28, respectively. The analyses are based on clustering 2100 independent components (100 ICA runs with 21 components in each run) into 21 clusters. In order to demonstrate the cluster quality to reflect the compactness and isolation of a cluster, an index of quality (*Iq*) is defined (Himberg *et al.*, 2004) as $Iq(k) = \bar{S}(k)_{int} - \bar{S}(k)_{ext}$. $\bar{S}(k)_{int}$ and $\bar{S}(k)_{ext}$ are the averages of the intra- and extra-cluster similarities, respectively. $k = 1, 2, \ldots, K$, and K is the number of clusters and is the number of components extracted by ICASSO. *Iq* ranges from zero to one. If *Iq* approaches one, the extraction of the corresponding component is stable and robust, which indicate the appearance of this common component in almost every run of the ICA decomposition. Otherwise, the component extracted by ICASSO is unstable, implying the occurrence of overfitting of that component (Himberg *et al.*, 2004; Vigario & Oja, 2008).

Figure 3.27 shows that the ICA decomposition results shown in Figure 3.25 are very stable because most *Iq*s approach one, and most clusters except one are isolated. This condition indicates some noisy components exist that do not belong to any good cluster. However, Figure 3.28 shows that the ICA decomposition results shown in Figure 3.26 are unstable because most clusters overlap. The clusters shown in Figures 3.27 and 3.28 are ranked according to decreasing cluster qualities.

Consequently, we accept the ICA decomposition results of the 21 principal components of the wavelet-filtered averaged EEG data and reject those of the ordinarily averaged EEG data. The example in this section also shows the benefit of appropriately designed wavelet filter.

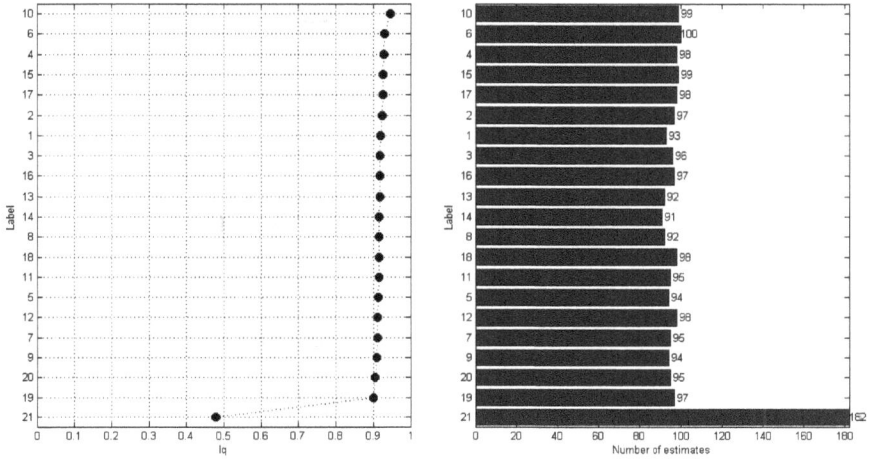

(a)

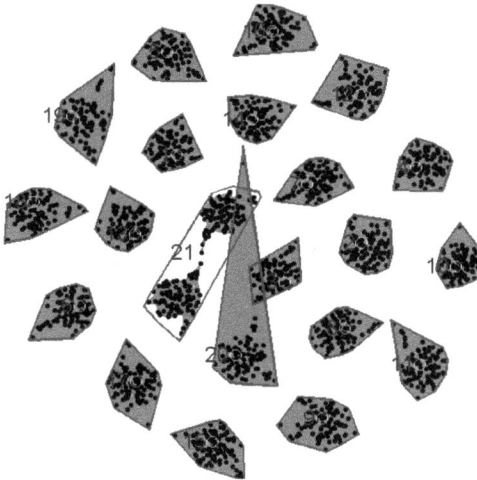

(b)

Figure 3.27   (a) Stability indexes of the independent components shown in Figure 3.25. (b) Clustering results of the 2100 independent components (100 runs with 21 components in each run) extracted by the ICA from the 21 PCA components of the wavelet-filtered averaged EEG data. Each dot in (b) represents one independent component.

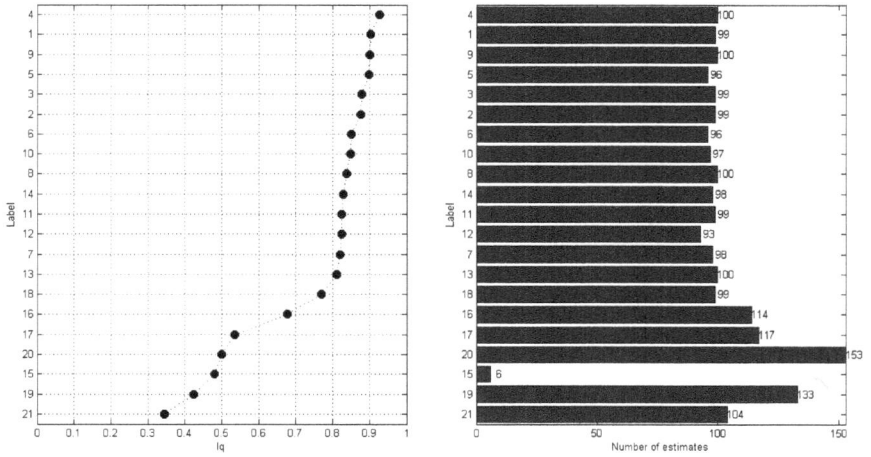

(a)

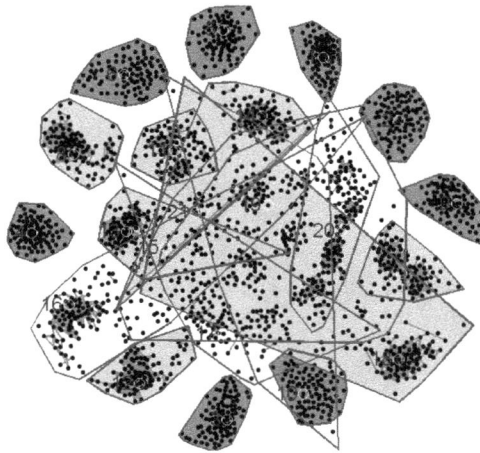

(b)

Figure 3.28   (a) Stability indexes of the independent components shown in Figure 3.26. (b) Clustering results of the 2100 independent components (100 runs with 21 components in each run) extracted by the ICA from the 21 PCA components of the ordinarily averaged EEG data. Each dot in (b) represents one independent component.

3.7.5 *Selection of the components of interest*

Because the experiment paradigm is to elicit MMN, the independent component of interest relevant to MMN should be selected among the 21 components shown in Figure 3.25. Two types of information are available for this task. One is the MMN latency, and the other is the MMN topography. They are introduced in the Appendix. Therefore, we select components #12 and #13 as the components of interest.

3.7.6 *Back-projection of selected components*

The variances and polarities of the independent components shown in Figure 3.25 are indeterminate. Therefore, they should be corrected before further analysis, which can be achieved in terms of Eq. (3-16), i.e.,

$$e_q(t) = \mathbf{V} \cdot \mathbf{b}_q \cdot y_q(t). \tag{3-40}$$

The dashed curve in Figure 3.23(a) shows the back-projection of independent components #12 and #13. By using the systematic ICA approach, the baseline becomes flat, and the ERP components irrelevant to MMN are removed.

The systematic ICA approach in extracting the ERP components from the averaged EEG data consists of six steps when they are collected by a high-density array.

3.8 Systematic ICA Approach to Extract the ERP Components from the Averaged EEG Data (DW) Collected by Low-Density Array

3.8.1 *Motivation*

The passive oddball paradigm is used to elicit the MMN, and difference wave (DW) is often used to study the MMN (Näätänen *et al.*, 2011, 2012). DW is based on the subtraction of the responses of the standard stimuli from those of the deviant stimuli. Therefore, knowing whether ICA can be applied to extract the MMN from the DW is interesting. We tried this idea in our previous study (Astikainen *et al.*, 2013). Because our previous study was not methodologically oriented, many details were not presented. Although the high-density array has been widely used to collect EEG data, the array that includes a few dozens of electrodes is still extensively applied in practice, particularly in clinical applications. Thus, knowing whether ICA can be applied to extract the ERP components from the averaged EEG data collected by a low-density array is also interesting.

3.8.2 *Introduction to DW*

In this section, we use the visual MMN (vMMN) example (Astikainen *et al.*, 2013; Astikainen & Hietanen, 2009; Astikainen, Lillstrang, & Ruusuvirta, 2008; Stefanics, Csukly, Komlosi, Czobor, & Czigler, 2012). The experimental paradigm is shown in Figure 1.1. After the preprocessing, the EEG data of approximately 100 single trials are averaged for each deviant stimulus (fearful/happy faces) and for each standard stimulus. Then, the average responses of the deviant stimulus is subtracted from the average responses of the standard stimulus, producing the DW (Astikainen *et al.*, 2013). The sampling frequency is 1000 Hz, the duration of one epoch is 700 ms (from −200 to 500 ms), and 14 electrodes are used for the data collection (Astikainen *et al.*, 2013). In this study, the DWs of one adult with a happy deviant stimulus are used for the demonstration. Figure 3.29(a) shows the DWs. Obviously, the DW is much noisier than the averaged responses to the stimuli (Kalyakin *et al.*, 2007).

3.8.3 *Six steps of the systematic ICA approach to extract the MMN component from the DW*

After the DW is produced, wavelet filtering is applied to filter the DW. The wavelet filter when the sampling frequency is 1000 Hz is shown in Figure 3.20. Then, the FastICA-based ICASSO is applied on the wavelet-filtered DW and the ordinarily averaged-based DW (hereinafter referred to as conventional DW). The FastICA is run 100 times, and 14 components are extracted in each runtime. Figures 3.30 and 3.31 show the independent components and their corresponding topographies, respectively, extracted from the wavelet-filtered and the conventional DWs. Obviously, the independent components from the wavelet-filtered DW are much cleaner, which again validates the analysis of Eq. (3-28). Figures 3.32 and 3.33 show the stability analyses of the independent components shown in Figures 3.30 and 3.31. The ICA decomposition on the wavelet-filtered DW is evidently

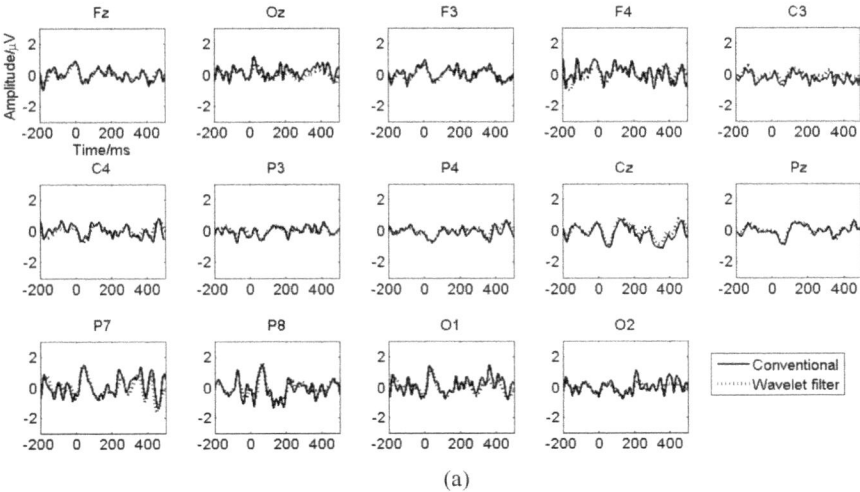

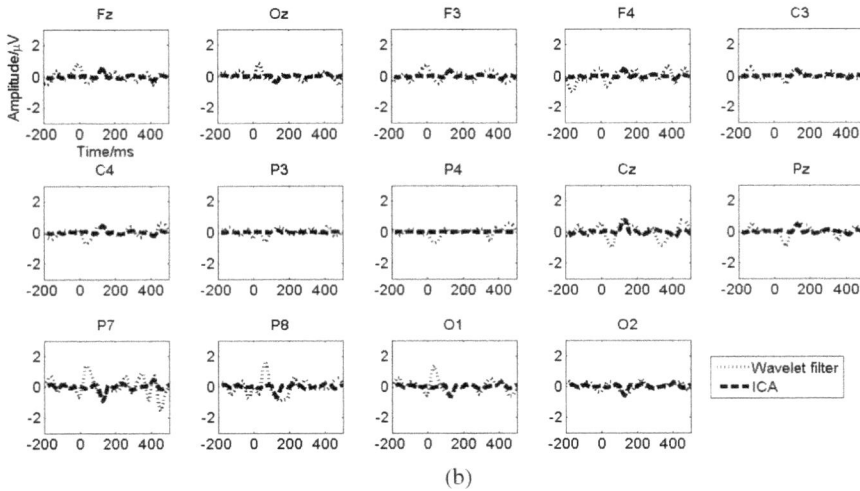

Figure 3.29 Waveforms of the DWs obtained by ordinary averaging, wavelet filtering, and systematic ICA approach. To clearly discriminate the different methods, the wavelet-filtered waveforms are plotted in both (a) and (b).

very stable, and that on the conventional DW is not stable at all. Component #14 is selected, and its back-projection is shown in Figure 3.29(b). Again, the systematic ICA approach removes the uninteresting components and makes the baseline flat.

(a)

(b)

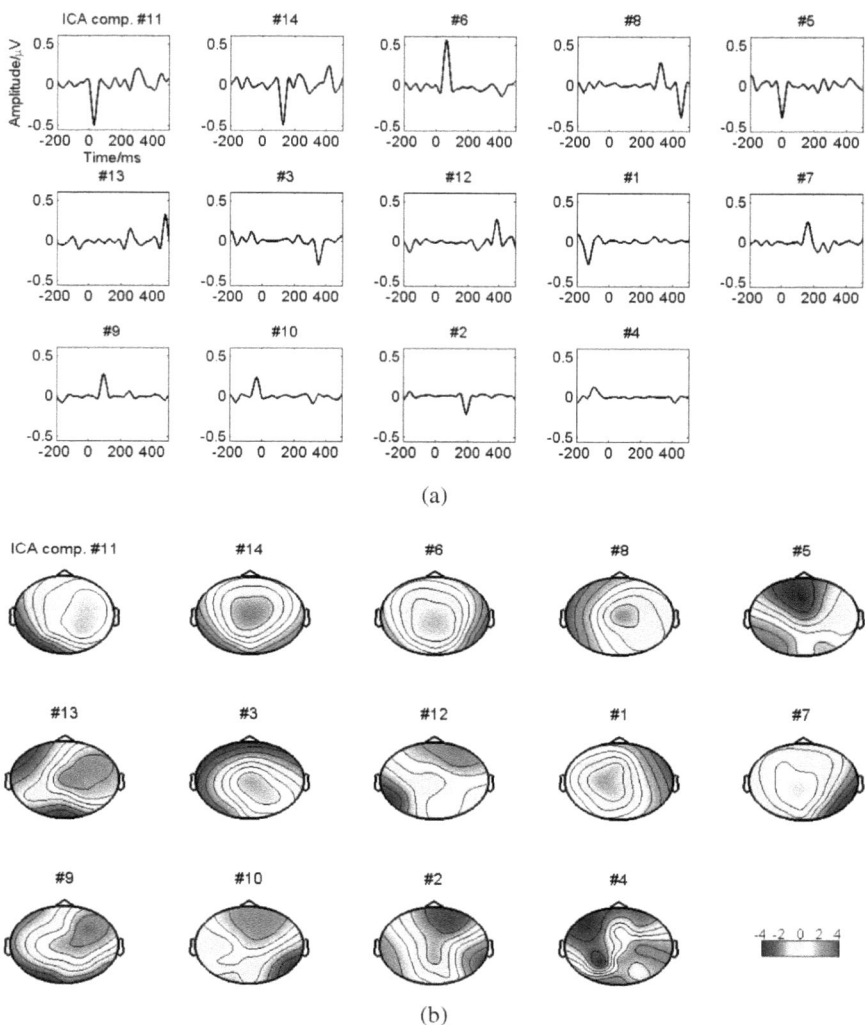

Figure 3.30 (a) Independent components extracted by the ICA from the wavelet-filtered DW shown in Figure 2.29. (b) Topographies of the independent components in (a). The variance and polarity of any component or topography are not determined in (a) and (b). The components are ordered according to their contributions to the mixture (Cong, Leppänen, *et al.*, 2011).

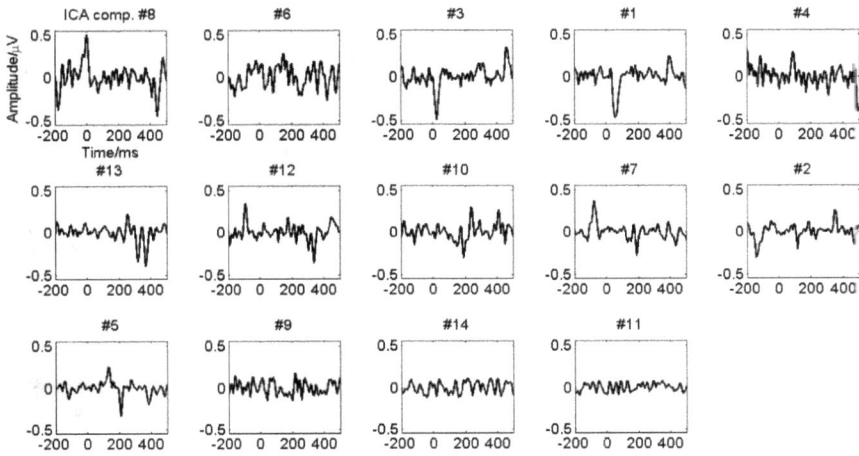

(a)

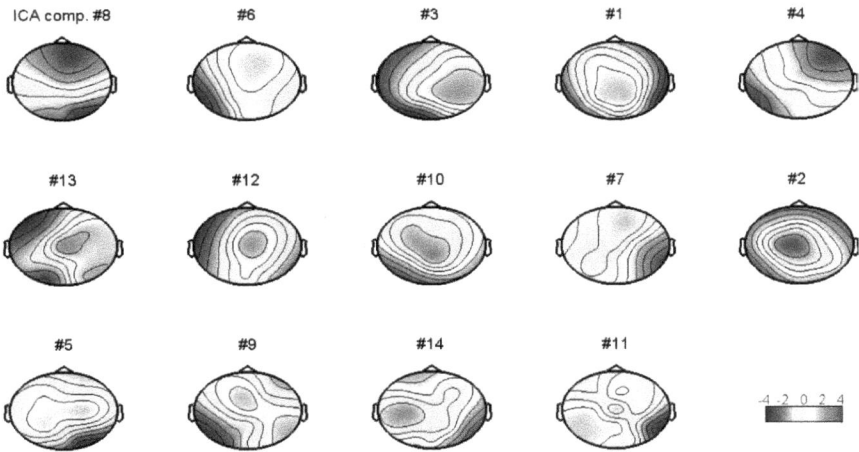

(b)

Figure 3.31 (a) Independent components extracted by the ICA from the ordinarily averaged-based DWs (i.e., conventional) shown in Figure 2.29. (b) Topographies of the independent components in (a). The variance and polarity of any component or topography are not determined in (a) and (b). The components are ordered according to their contributions to the mixture (Cong, Leppänen, *et al.*, 2011).

(a)

(b)

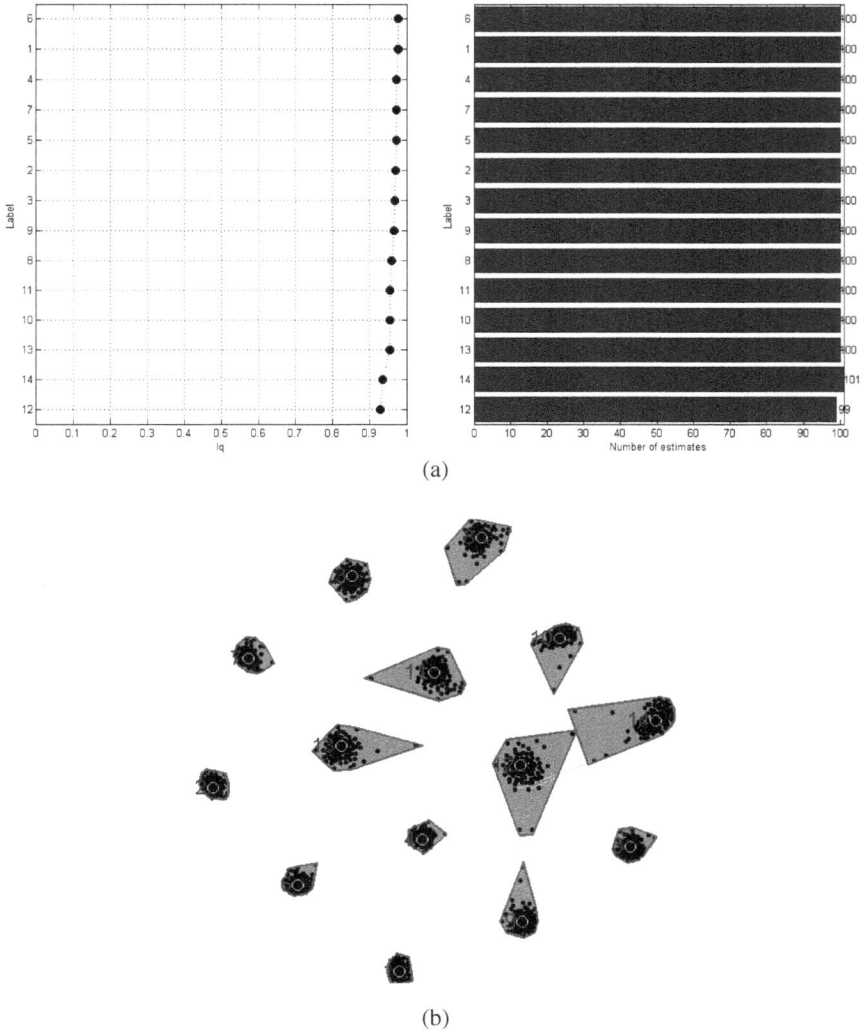

Figure 3.32   (a) Stability indexes of the independent components shown in Figure 3.30. (b) Clustering results of the 1400 independent components (100 runs with 14 components in each run) extracted by the ICA from the wavelet-filtered DWs shown in Figure 3.29. Each dot in (b) represents one independent component.

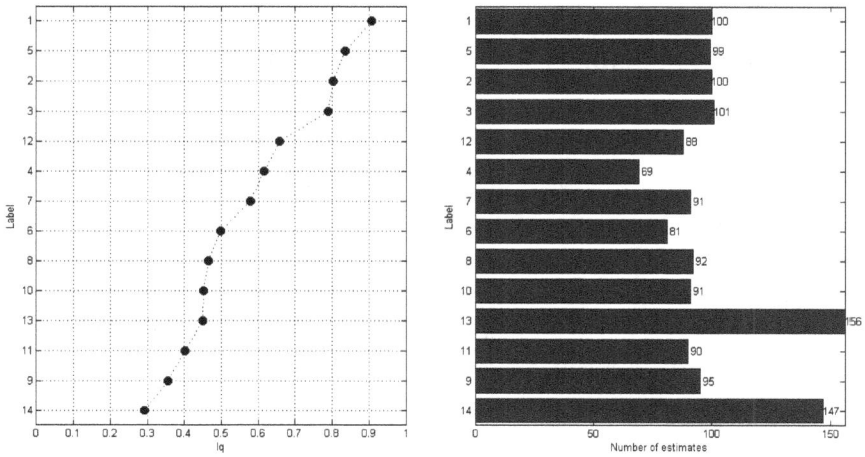

(a)

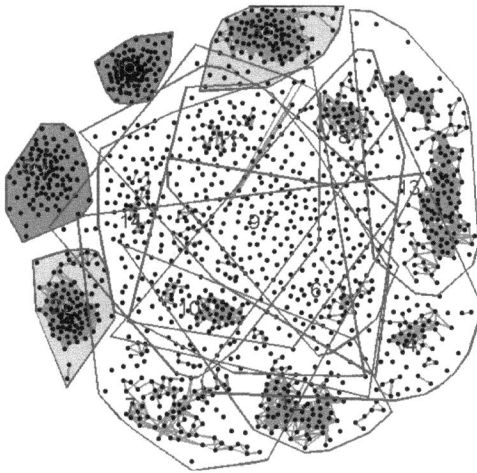

(b)

Figure 3.33   (a) Stability indexes of the independent components shown in Figure 3.31. (b) Clustering results of the 1400 independent components (100 runs with 14 components in each run) extracted by the ICA from the ordinarily averaged-based DWs shown in Figure 3.29. Each dot in (b) represents one independent component.

3.9 Reliability of the Independent Components Extracted by the Systematic ICA Approach from Averaged EEG Data

Nowadays, when ICA is applied on the EEG data, it is usually performed on concatenated single-trial EEG data. This has been taught in the EEGLAB workshop since the 2000s. Many learning materials can be accessed via http://sccn.ucsd.edu/wiki/EEGLAB. With the development of EEGLAB, an increasing number of researchers have studied ICA for EEG data processing. We should note that the concatenated single-trial EEG data are very long. As a result, when ICA is applied on the averaged EEG data, we often encounter such comment as "You do not have enough data for ICA decomposition to extract the independent components." Indeed, irrespective of how ICA is applied on which type of EEG data, success of the ICA decomposition on the EEG data cannot be achieved unless the six steps listed in Section 3.7 are very well implemented. In this section, we further present the reasons why the independent components extracted by our systematic ICA approach from the averaged EEG data are reliable.

3.9.1 *Simulation study: Sufficiency of several hundreds of samples in extracting a few dozens of sources*

In the early years of ICA, simulation study was required to demonstrate the superiority of the proposed ICA algorithm over the existing ICA algorithms (Cichocki & Amari, 2003; Comon & Jutten, 2010; Hyvarinen *et al.*, 2001). When ICA is applied to decompose the EEG data, a similar simulation study is difficult to perform because we do not know the true sources and cannot evaluate the performance of a certain ICA algorithm on the basis of the true sources and mixing matrices (Cichocki & Amari, 2003; Comon & Jutten, 2010; Hyvarinen *et al.*, 2001). In this book, we do not compare the performance of the different algorithms. The purpose of the simulation here is to show that we successfully extract 14 sources from the mixtures using ICASSO when 14-channel mixtures are collected with each channel containing only 700 samples.

Figure 3.34(a) shows the 14 sources. They are independent components extracted by the systematic ICA approach. The full-rank mixing matrix with

(a)

(b)

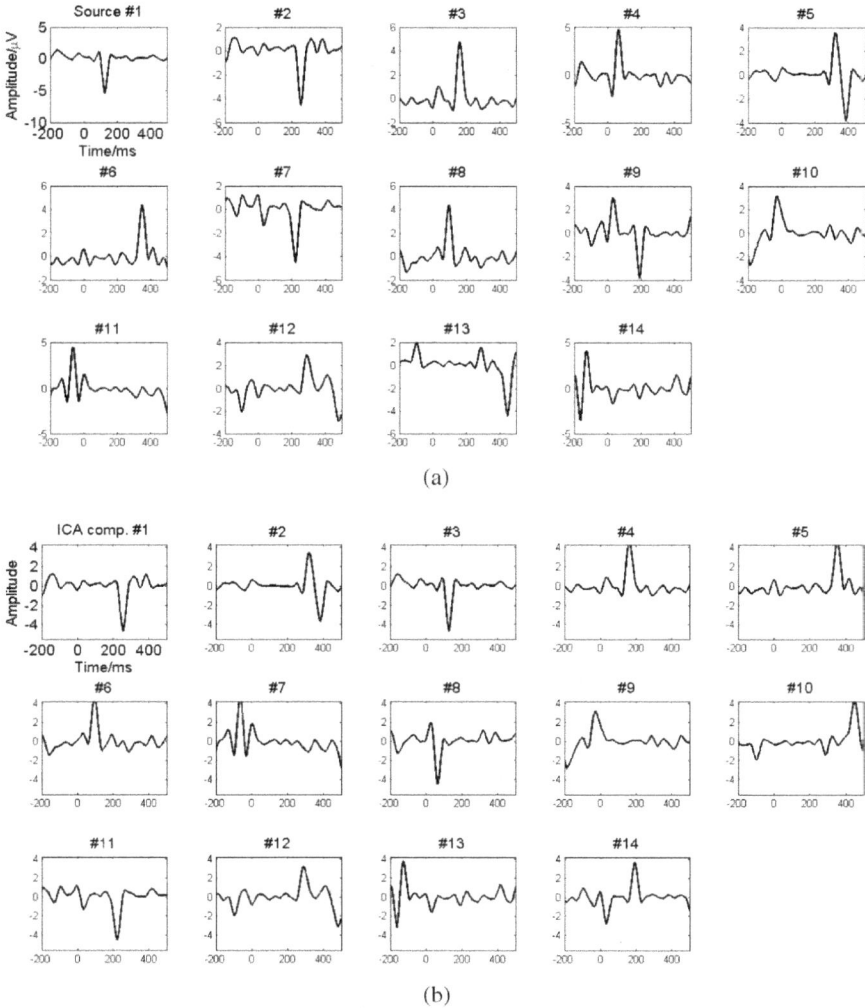

Figure 3.34 (a) 14 sources. (b) 14 independent components extracted by ICA from the simulated mixtures. The simulation is performed on the basis of Eq. (3.6), and the mixing matrix is randomly generated. The variances and polarities are not determined in (b).

a size of 14×14 is randomly generated. Then, the 14-channel mixtures are simulated according to Eq. (3-6). The FastICA-based ICASSO is applied to extract the 14 independent components shown in Figure 3.34(b). The extracted components are very similar to the sources.

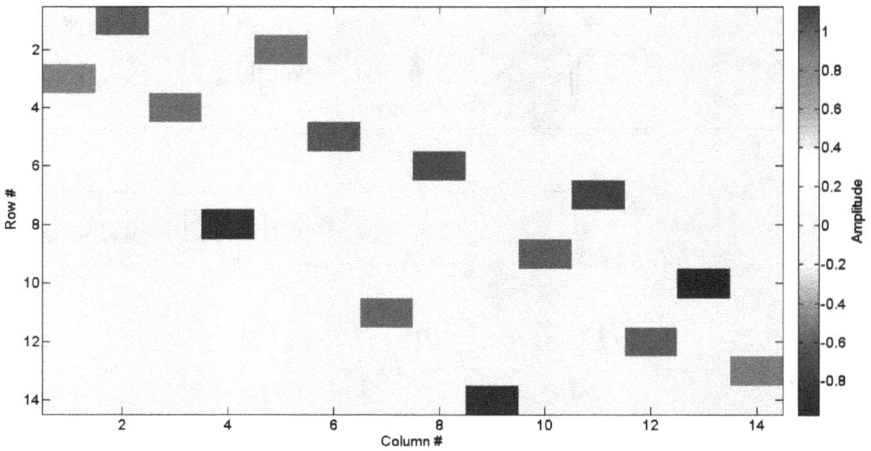

Figure 3.35 Global matrix of the satisfactory ICA decomposition in extracting the components shown in Figure 3.35. In each row and column, one element has a much bigger absolute value than any other elements in that row and column.

Here, because the mixing and unmixing matrices are known, the global matrix is available in terms of Eq. (3-11). Figure 3.35 shows the global matrix. Obviously, only one element exists with a relatively much bigger amplitude in each row and column than any other elements in that row and column. This result indicates that the ICA decomposition is very successful (Cong, Kalyakin, & Ristaniemi, 2011; Cong, Kalyakin, Zheng, *et al.*, 2011).

This example demonstrates that 700 samples are sufficient to extract the 14 sources when the mixtures meet the assumptions of the ICA algorithm and the ICA model.

3.9.2 *Are bump-like independent components reasonable when the systematic ICA approach is applied on the averaged EEG data?*

When the systematic ICA approach is applied, bump-like components can be extracted similar to those shown in Figures 3.25(a) and 3.30(a). These components appear very different from the independent components extracted from the concatenated single trials shown in Figure 3.7. Therefore, we need to decide whether the bump-like components are reasonable or not.

First, two components (#12 and #13) relative to MMN are selected, as shown in Figure 3.25(a). After they are projected back to the electrode field, the back-projection shown in Figure 3.23(a) appears similar to the normal ERP component, which means that two or more independent components may belong to one ERP component. Indeed, when the discrete model is used for EEG/magnetoencephalography (MEG) source localization, a few dipoles are often used (Hämäläinen, Ortiz-Mantilla, & Benasich, 2011; Hämäläinen, Rupp, Soltesz, Szucs, & Goswami, 2012; Ortiz-Mantilla, Hämäläinen, & Benasich, 2012; Ortiz-Mantilla, Hämäläinen, Musacchia, & Benasich, 2013). Therefore, it is reasonable that one ERP component can reasonably correspond to a few independent components extracted by the systematic ICA approach.

Second, the systematic ICA approach very stably extracts the bump-like components, as shown in Figures 3.27 and 3.32. Vigario and Oja stated that if the bump-like components are technical artifacts produced by overfitting, they cannot be stably extracted (Vigario & Oja, 2008). Therefore, we can reasonably conclude that the bump-like components are linked to the real ERP component when the systematic ICA approach is applied.

Finally, the topography of an independent component is very important in determining whether the component is reliable or not. Recently, the independent component has been concluded to be dipolar (Cong, Alluri, *et al.*, 2013; Delorme *et al.*, 2012; Lin, Duann, Feng, Chen, & Jung, 2014). Therefore, if the topography is locally focused like most of the topographies shown in Figure 3.25(b), the underlying brain activity may be correct. If the topography is scattered, it may belong to technical artifacts. Because most of the topographies of the independent components extracted by the systematic ICA approach are reasonable in Figure 3.25(b), we can conclude that the ICA decomposition shown in Figure 3.25 is successful, and the extracted components are reasonable.

3.10 Benefits of the Wavelet Filter in the Systematic ICA Approach to Extract the ERP Components from Averaged EEG Data

In this study, appropriately designing the wavelet filter is an ICA preprocess. The clustering results shown in Figures 3.22, 3.23, 3.27, and 3.28 clearly demonstrate the usefulness of the wavelet filters. For the 14-channel data, the difference in the results shown in Figures 3.22 and 3.23 lies in the usage of the wavelet filter. After the wavelet filter is applied, the ICA decomposition becomes stable, allowing the ICA to successfully extract the ERP components. Such success results from the two benefits (explained below) gained from the appropriately designed wavelet filter.

One of the benefits is that the wavelet filter denoises the noisy sources. Equation (3-28) illustrates that, in practice, real ICA sources are noisy and not noise-free, as shown in Figures 3.25(a), 3.26(a), 3.30(a), and 3.31(a). Denoising the noisy sources lets the ICA more effectively exploit the independence among the noise-free sources.

The other benefit is that the wavelet filter reduces the number of sources (Cong, He, *et al.*, 2013; Cong, Leppänen, *et al.*, 2011). Figure 3.23(b) shows that many sources are removed, which reduces the complexity of the next ICA decomposition (Karhunen, Hao, & Ylipaavalniemi, 2013) and converts the under-determined model into a determined model. For example, for the 14-channel DWs shown in Figure 3.29(a), the linear transform model of the DWs is certainly under-determined because the number of sources is surely much bigger than 14. When the determined ICA algorithm (14-source–14-channel–14-component) is implemented, the ICA decomposition becomes unstable, as shown in Figure 3.33. This is because the model of the data to be decomposed and that of the ICA algorithm do not match. In other words, the 14-channel DWs cannot be modeled by the 14-source–14-channel linear transform model. After the wavelet filtering, the ICA decomposition becomes surprisingly stable, as shown in Figure 3.32, indicating that the wavelet-filtered 14-channel DWs can be modeled by the 14-source–14-channel linear transform model.

3.11 Relationship among the Global Optimization of the ICA Decomposition, Stability of the ICA Decomposition, ICA Algorithm, and Number of Extracted Components

Section 3.2.2.2 mentioned that no indeterminacy exists in the decomposed results when the ICA decomposition reaches the global optimization. However, obtaining the global optimization in practice is not realistic

(Himberg *et al.*, 2004). When the ICA decomposition is stable and the extracted independent components and their topographies are meaningful, we consider that the decomposition is very close to the global optimization; otherwise, obtaining such results is very difficult.

In practice, two factors can affect the stability of the ICA decomposition. One is the ICA algorithm, which has been very extensively acknowledged, and the other is the number of components extracted by the ICA. Given a dataset and an ICA algorithm, the algorithm may converge when different numbers of components are tried. Indeed, the number of true sources is fixed in a given dataset. However, one dataset can be modeled by different linear transform models with different numbers of sources. The number of sources tends to be smaller than the number of true sources, and the sources partially overlap the true sources. When ICA is applied to decompose the EEG data, noisy components are inevitable (Delorme *et al.*, 2012), and the noisy components are a mixture of some true sources and noise. As mentioned earlier, as long as the "ICA decomposition is stable and the extracted independent components and their topographies are meaningful," the ICA decomposition on the EEG data is successful, and the linear transform model with a selected number of components is appropriate to model the EEG data.

3.12 Summary

ICA can be regarded as a spatial filter, which is illustrated in Eqs. (3-14) and (3-24). The systematic ICA approach sequentially filters the ERP data (averaged EEG) in the time, frequency, and space domains. To extract the ERP components of a subject under one condition using ICA, we recommend applying individual ICA on the averaged EEG data based on a systematic approach, which includes the following steps:

(1) The single-trial EEG data are preprocessed, and the preprocessed EEG data are averaged over single trials.
(2) The averaged EEG data are filtered using an appropriately designed wavelet filter (please see Section 3.6.3.2).
(3) The number of sources in the wavelet-filtered averaged EEG data is estimated, and the over-determined model is converted into the

determined model when a high-density array is used to collect the EEG data (please see Section 3.5).

(4) The FastICA-based ICASSO is implemented on the data of the determined model to extract the independent components. If the ICA decomposition is not stable, the decomposed results are not accepted for further analysis, and the second and third steps are repeated. If the ICA decomposition is stable, the decomposed results are accepted for further analysis, and the next step is performed.

(5) The independent components of interest are selected according to the latency and topography of the ERP component.

(6) The selected independent components are projected back to the electrode field to correct the variance and polarity indeterminacies of the independent components. At any typical electrode of the ERP, if the amplitude of the ERP back-projection becomes abnormally large or small or the polarity is reversed, the results are not accepted, and data processing is run again (Cong, Kalyakin, & Ristaniemi, 2011; Cong, Kalyakin, Zheng, *et al.*, 2011).

We should note that the data to be decomposed in Step (4) may be upsampled a few times to obtain enough number of samples for the ICA decomposition. After the ICA decomposition, the extracted independent components are downsampled back to the original sampling frequency. Because the EEG data are usually uniformly sampled and possess very high time resolution and the sampling algorithm is very accurate, up- and downsampling a few times do not cause dark effects on the systematic ICA approach on the averaged EEG data.

3.13 Existing Key Problems and Potential Solutions

Sections 3.6.4 and 3.7.4 introduced that the stability of the ICA decomposition on the ERP data is based on the clustering of the extracted independent temporal components from multiple runs. Indeed, Figure 1.3 shows that a source includes a temporal and a spatial component (i.e., topography). If the temporal components are stably extracted, we still do not know whether the spatial components are stably extracted or not. Therefore, to thoroughly investigate the stability of the ICA decomposition, both the temporal and spatial components should be used in the clustering.

Furthermore, when a high-density array is used in the EEG data collection, dimension reduction by the PCA can produce some technical artifacts owing to the inherent orthogonal constraints. The technical artifacts can affect the stability of the next ICA decomposition. Figure 3.27 shows that one cluster is not sufficient. When the EEG source localization is not the research interest, including hundreds of sensors in the ICA is unnecessary because the number of sources can only be a few dozens after the appropriate wavelet filter is applied. Therefore, we can simply choose as many channel data as the number of sources for the ICA decomposition. The selected channels should be more representative of the ERP of interest among all channels.

3.14 MATLAB Codes

3.14.1 *Systematic ICA approach on averaged EEG data collected by high-density array*

Please note that ICASSO and FastICA toolboxes are used. You may download ICASSO via http://research.ics.aalto.fi/ica/icasso/ and FastICA via link http://research.ics.aalto.fi/ica/fastica/. In order to plot the topography of an independent component, the "topoplot" function in EEGLAB should be used as well as the coordinates of electrodes. EEGLAB can be downloaded via http://sccn.ucsd.edu/eeglab/. Demo data can be accessed via http://www.escience.cn/people/cong/index.html.

In order to use those toolboxes and the demo data, one has to know how to program with MATLAB. The core function for the systematic ICA approach is as the following:

```
function [Y,TOPO,Iq] = f_systematicICA_highDenseEEG(x,fs)
%%% input
%%%%%%%% x: Averaged EEG data with the sizes of M channels by
T samples
%%%%%%%% fs: sampling frequency of the signal
%%% output
%%%%%%%% Y: extracted independent components
%%%%%%%% TOPO: topographies of independent components
%%%%%%%% Iq: index of quality of stability of ICA decompostion
%%
```

```
[NumChannels, NumSamps] = size(x);
%% wavelet filter
wname= 'rbio6.8'; %%% name of the wavelet
switch 1
    case fs == 1000
    lv=10; %% number of levels for the decomposition
    kp=[9 8 7 6]; %% the coefficients at the levels 9, 8, 7, and 6 are chosen
for the reconstruction
    case fs == 500
    lv=9; %% number of levels for the decomposition
    kp=[8 7 6 5]; %% the coefficients at the levels 8, 7, 6, and 5 are chosen
for the reconstruction
    case fs <500
    lv=8; %% number of levels for the decomposition
    kp=[7 6 5 4]; %% the coefficients at the levels 7, 6, 5, and 4 are chosen
for the reconstruction
end
for is = 1:NumChannels
    X(is,:) = f_filterWavelet(x(is,:),lv,wname,kp);
end
%% Determining the number of sources
[Vx,Z,lambda] = princomp(X');
%%% estimate the number of sources in the noisy mixtures through model
order selection-GAP
R = f_Gap(lambda,eps);
%% dimension reduction, i.e., converting overdetermined model to deter-
mined model
V = Vx(:,1:R);
SelectedPCAcomponents = Z(:,1:R);
ratio = 4;
SelectedPCAcomponents = resample(SelectedPCAcomponents,ratio,1);
%%% upsampling the data to have more samples for avoiding overfitting
in ICA decomposition
%% ICASSO
```

```
NumSources = R;
NumRuns = 100;
sR =icassoEst('both', SelectedPCAcomponents', NumRuns, 'numOfIC',
NumSources, 'g', 'tanh', 'approach', 'symm');
sRExp=icassoExp(sR);
[Iq,A,W,S]=icassoShow(sRExp,'L',NumSources,'colorlimit',[.8 .9]);
Y = resample(S',1,ratio); %%% downsampling to the original sampling
frequency when the data was imported
Y = Y';
TOPO = V*A;
```

3.14.2 *Model order selection*

```
function R=f_Gap(lambda, eps)
%% MATLAB codes for GAP were written by Professor Zhaoshui He
%% in Guangdong University of Technology, Guang Zhou, China
%% Email: he_shui@tom.com
%% Reference: Z. He, A. Cichocki, S. Xie and K. Choi,
%% Detecting the number of clusters in n-way probabilistic clustering
%% IEEE Trans. Pattern Anal. Mach. Intell., 32: 2006-2021, 2010
%% %%% input: lambda represents eigenvalues
len=length(lambda);
nklambda=sort(lambda,1,'descend');
for k=0:len-1
    if (k<len-2)
    temp=mean(nklambda(k+2:len));
    if (nklambda(k+1)-temp<eps)
    GAP(k+1)=1;
    else
    GAP(k+1)=(nklambda(k+2)-temp)/(nklambda(k+1)-temp);
    end
    end
end
[kkvalue,R]=min(GAP);
```

3.14.3 *Systematic ICA approach on averaged EEG data collected by low-density array*

The demonstration of MATLAB codes and ERP data of 14 channels can be found from the supplementary material of our previous paper (Astikainen *et al.*, 2013). The link is as the following:

http://journal.frontiersin.org/Journal/10.3389/fnhum.2013.00557/abstract

References

Abou-Elseoud, A., Starck, T., Remes, J., Nikkinen, J., Tervonen, O., & Kiviniemi, V. (2010). The effect of model order selection in group PICA. *Human Brain Mapping*, *31*(8), 1207–1216. doi: 10.1002/hbm.20929.

Akaike, H. (1974). A new look at statistical model identification. *IEEE Transactions on Automatic Control*, *19*, 716–723.

Alkhaldi, W., Iskander, D. R., & Zoubir, A. M. (2010). Improving the performance of model-order selection criteria by partial-model selection search. Paper presented at the 2010 *IEEE International Conference on Acoustics Speech and Signal Processing (ICASSP2010)*.

Astikainen, P., Cong, F., Ristaniemi, T., & Hietanen, J. K. (2013). Event-related potentials to unattended changes in facial expressions: Detection of regularity violations or encoding of emotions? *Frontiers in Human Neuroscience*, *7*, 557. doi: 10.3389/fnhum.2013.00557; 10.3389/fnhum.2013.00557.

Astikainen, P. & Hietanen, J. K. (2009). Event-related potentials to task-irrelevant changes in facial expressions. *Behavioral and Brain Functions: BBF*, *5*, 30. doi: 10.1186/1744-9081-5-30.

Astikainen, P., Lillstrang, E., & Ruusuvirta, T. (2008). Visual mismatch negativity for changes in orientation — A sensory memory-dependent response. *The European Journal of Neuroscience*, *28*(11), 2319–2324. doi: 10.1111/j.1460-9568.2008.06510.x.

Beckmann, C. F. & Smith, S. M. (2004). Probabilistic independent component analysis for functional magnetic resonance imaging. *IEEE Transactions on Medical Imaging*, *23*(2), 137–152. doi: 10.1109/TMI.2003.822821.

Bishop, C. M. (2006). *Pattern Recognition and Machine Learning* (Vol. 1). Singapore: Springer.

Bishop, D. V. & Hardiman, M. J. (2010). Measurement of mismatch negativity in individuals: A study using single-trial analysis. *Psychophysiology*, *47*(4), 697–705. doi: 10.1111/j.1469-8986.2009.00970.x.

Cavanaugh, J. E. (1999). A large-sample model selection criterion based on Kullback's symmetric divergence. *Statistics & Probability Letters*, *44*, 333–344.

Cichocki, A. & Amari, S. (2003). *Adaptive Blind Signal and Image Processing: Learning Algorithms and Applications* (Vol. Revised). Chichester: John Wiley & Sons Inc.

Comon, P. (1994). Independent component analysis, a new concept? *Signal Processing*, *36*(3), 287–314.

Comon, P. & Jutten, C. (2010). *Handbook of Blind Source Separation: Independent Component Analysis and Applications* (Vol. 1). Academic Press.

Comon, P., Jutten, C., & Herault, J. (1991). Blind separation of sources, Part II: Problems statement. *Signal Processing*, *24*(1), 11–20.

Cong, F., Alluri, V., Nandi, A. K., Toiviainen, P., Fa, R., Abu-Jamous, B., ... Ristaniemi, T. (2013). Linking brain responses to naturalistic music through analysis of ongoing EEG and stimulus features. *IEEE Transactions on Multimedia*, *15*(5), 1060–1069.

Cong, F., He, Z., Hämäläinen, J., Cichocki, A., & Ristaniemi, T. (2011). Determining the number of sources in high-density EEG recordings of event-related potentials by model order selection. *Proceedings of IEEE Workshop on Machine Learning for Signal Processing (MLSP) 2011*, Beijing, China, September 18–21, 1–6.

Cong, F., He, Z., Hämäläinen, J., Leppänen, P. H. T., Lyytinen, H., Cichocki, A., & Ristaniemi, T. (2013). Validating rationale of group-level component analysis based on estimating number of sources in EEG through model order selection. *Journal of Neuroscience Methods*, *212*(1), 165–172.

Cong, F., Kalyakin, I., Ahuttunen-Scott, T., Li, H., Lyytinen, H., & Ristaniemi, T. (2010). Single-trial based independent component analysis on mismatch negativity in children. *International Journal of Neural Systems*, *20*(4), 279–292.

Cong, F., Kalyakin, I., Li, H., Huttunen-Scott, T., Huang, Y. X., Lyytinen, H., & Ristaniemi, T. (2011). Answering six questions in extracting children's mismatch negativity through combining wavelet decomposition and independent component analysis. *Cognitive Neurodynamics*, *5*(4), 343–359.

Cong, F., Kalyakin, I., & Ristaniemi, T. (2011). Can back-projection fully resolve polarity indeterminacy of ICA in study of ERP? *Biomedical Signal Processing and Control*, *6*(4), 422–426.

Cong, F., Kalyakin, I., Zheng, C., & Ristaniemi, T. (2011). Analysis on subtracting projection of extracted independent components from EEG recordings. *Biomedizinische Technik/Biomedical Engineering*, *56*(4), 223–234.

Cong, F., Leppänen, P. H., Astikainen, P., Hämäläinen, J., Hietanen, J. K., & Ristaniemi, T. (2011). Dimension reduction: Additional benefit of an optimal filter for independent component analysis to extract event-related potentials. *Journal of Neuroscience Methods*, *201*(1), 269–280. doi: 10.1016/j.jneumeth.2011.07.015.

Cong, F., Nandi, A. K., He, Z., Cichocki, A., & Ristaniemi, T. (2012). Fast and effective model order selection method to determine the number of sources in a linear transformation model. *Proceedings of the 2012 European Signal Processing Conference (EUSIPCO-2012)*, 1870–1874.

Cong, F., Puolivali, T., Alluri, V., Sipola, T., Burunat, I., Toiviainen, P., ... Ristaniemi, T. (2014). Key issues in decomposing fMRI during naturalistic and continuous music experience with independent component analysis. *Journal of Neuroscience Methods*, *223*, 74–84. doi: 10.1016/j.jneumeth.2013.11.025.

Cong, F. & Ristaniemi, T. (2011). Data model conversion for independent component analysis to extract brain signals. *Proceedings of IEEE 3rd International Conference on Awareness Science and Technology 2011*, Dalian, China, September 27–30, 188–193.

Delorme, A. & Makeig, S. (2004). EEGLAB: An open source toolbox for analysis of single-trial EEG dynamics including independent component analysis. *Journal of Neuroscience Methods*, *134*(1), 9–21. doi: 10.1016/j.jneumeth.2003.10.009.

Delorme, A., Palmer, J., Onton, J., Oostenveld, R., & Makeig, S. (2012). Independent EEG sources are dipolar. *PloS One*, *7*(2), e30135. doi: 10.1371/journal.pone.0030135.

Eichele, T., Rachakonda, S., Brakedal, B., Eikeland, R., & Calhoun, V. D. (2011). EEGIFT: Group independent component analysis for event-related EEG data. *Computational Intelligence and Neuroscience*, *2011*, 129365. doi: 10.1155/2011/129365.

Groppe, D. M., Makeig, S., & Kutas, M. (2009). Identifying reliable independent components via split-half comparisons. *NeuroImage*, *45*(4), 1199–1211. doi: 10.1016/j.neuroimage.2008.12.038.

Hämäläinen, J., Ortiz-Mantilla, S., & Benasich, A. (2011). Source localization of event-related potentials to pitch change mapped onto age-appropriate MRIs at 6 months-of-age. *NeuroImage*, *54*(3), 1910–1918.

Hämäläinen, J., Rupp, A., Soltesz, F., Szucs, D., & Goswami, U. (2012). Reduced phase locking to slow amplitude modulation in adults with dyslexia: An MEG study. *Neuroimage*, *59*(3), 2952–2961.

Hansen, M. H. & Yu, B. (2001). Model selection and the principle of minimum description length. *Journal of the American Statistical Association*, *96*(154), 746–774.

He, Z., Cichocki, A., Xie, S., & Choi, K. (2010). Detecting the number of clusters in n-way probabilistic clustering. *IEEE Transactions on Pattern Analysis and Machine Intelligence*, *32*(11), 2006–2021. doi: 10.1109/TPAMI.2010.15.

He, Z. S., Cichocki, A., & Xie, S. (2009). Efficient method for Tucker3 model selection. *Electronics Letters*, *45*(15), 805–806.

Himberg, J., Hyvarinen, A., & Esposito, F. (2004). Validating the independent components of neuroimaging time series via clustering and visualization. *NeuroImage*, *22*(3), 1214–1222. doi: 10.1016/j.neuroimage.2004.03.027.

Hyvarinen, A. (1999). Fast and robust fixed-point algorithms for independent component analysis. *IEEE Transactions on Neural Networks/A Publication of the IEEE Neural Networks Council*, *10*(3), 626–634. doi: 10.1109/72.761722.

Hyvarinen, A. (2011). Testing the ICA mixing matrix based on inter-subject or inter-session consistency. *NeuroImage*, *58*(1), 122–136. doi: 10.1016/j.neuroimage.2011.05.086; 10.1016/j.neuroimage.2011.05.086.

Hyvarinen, A. (2013). Independent component analysis: Recent advances. *Proceedings of the Royal Society A: Mathematical, Physical, and Engineering Sciences*, *371*(20110534), 1–19. doi: 10.1098/rsta.2011.0534.

Hyvarinen, A., Karhunen, J., & Oja, E. (2001). *Independent Component Analysis*. New York: John Wiley & Sons Inc.

Hyvarinen, A. & Ramkumar, P. (2013). Testing independent component patterns by inter-subject or inter-session consistency. *Frontiers in Human Neuroscience*, *7*, 94. doi: 10.3389/fnhum.2013.00094.

Iyer, D. & Zouridakis, G. (2007). Single-trial evoked potential estimation: Comparison between independent component analysis and wavelet denoising. *Clinical Neurophysiology: Official Journal of the International Federation of Clinical Neurophysiology*, *118*(3), 495–504. doi: 10.1016/j.clinph.2006.10.024.

Jolliffe, I. (2002). *Principal Component Analysis* (Vol. 2). New York: Springer-Verlag.

Jung, T. P., Makeig, S., Humphries, C., Lee, T. W., McKeown, M. J., Iragui, V., & Sejnowski, T. J. (2000). Removing electroencephalographic artifacts by blind source separation. *Psychophysiology*, *37*(2), 163–178.

Jung, T. P., Makeig, S., Westerfield, M., Townsend, J., Courchesne, E., & Sejnowski, T. J. (2000). Removal of eye activity artifacts from visual event-related potentials in normal and clinical subjects. *Clinical Neurophysiology: Official Journal of the International Federation of Clinical Neurophysiology, 111*(10), 1745–1758.

Jutten, C. & Herault, J. (1991). Blind separation of sources, part I: An adaptive algorithm based on neuromimetic architecture. *Signal Processing, 24*(1), 1–10.

Kalyakin, I., Gonzalez, M., Ivannikov, I., & Lyytinen, H. (2009). Extraction of the mismatch negativity elicited by sound duration decrements: A comparison of three procedures. *Data & Knowledge Engineering, 68*(12), 1411–1426.

Kalyakin, I., Gonzalez, N., Joutsensalo, J., Huttunen, T., Kaartinen, J., & Lyytinen, H. (2007). Optimal digital filtering versus difference waves on the mismatch negativity in an uninterrupted sound paradigm. *Developmental Neuropsychology, 31*(3), 429–452. doi: 10.1080/87565640701229607.

Kalyakin, I., Gonzalez, N., Kärkkäinen, T., & Lyytinen, H. (2008). Independent component analysis on the mismatch negativity in an uninterrupted sound paradigm. *Journal of Neuroscience Methods, 174*(2), 301–312. doi: 10.1016/j.jneumeth.2008.07.012.

Karhunen, J., Hao, T., & Ylipaavalniemi, J. (2013). Finding dependent and independent components from related data sets: A generalized canonical correlation based method. *Neurocomputing, 113*, 153–167.

Kay, S. M., Nuttall, A. H., & Baggenstoss, P. M. (2001). Multidimensional probability density function approximations for detection, classification, and model order selection. *IEEE Transactions on Signal Processing, 49*(10), 2240–2252.

Kovacevic, N. & McIntosh, A. R. (2007). Groupwise independent component decomposition of EEG data and partial least square analysis. *NeuroImage, 35*(3), 1103–1112. doi 10.1016/j.neuroimage.2007.01.016.

Landi, N. (2012). *The Sixth Conference on Mismatch Negativity (MMN) and its Clinical and Scientific Application 2012.* City University of New York (CUNY), New York, USA, Abstract.

Li, Y. O., Adali, T., & Calhoun, V. D. (2007). Estimating the number of independent components for functional magnetic resonance imaging data. *Human Brain Mapping, 28*(11), 1251–1266. doi: 10.1002/hbm.20359.

Liavas, A. P. & Regalia, P. A. (2001). On the behavior of information theoretic criteria for model order selection. *IEEE Transactions on Signal Processing, 49*(8), 1689–1695.

Liavas, A. P., Regalia, P. A., & Delmas, J. P. (1999). Blind channel approximation: Effective channel order determination. *IEEE Transactions on Signal Processing, 47*(12). 3336–3344.

Lin, Y. P., Duann, J. R., Feng, W. F., Chen, J. H., & Jung, T. P. (2014). Revealing spatio-spectral electroencephalographic dynamics of musical mode and tempo perception by independent component analysis. *Journal of NeuroEngineering and Rehabilitation. 11*(18), 1–11.

Lindsen, J. P. & Bhattacharya, J. (2010). Correction of blink artifacts using independent component analysis and empirical mode decomposition. *Psychophysiology, 47*(5). 955–960. doi: 10.1111/j.1469-8986.2010.00995.x.

Lozano-Soldevilla, D., Marco-Pallares, J., Fuentemilla, L., & C., Grau. (2012). Common N1 and mismatch negativity neural evoked components are revealed by independent component model-based clustering analysis. *Psychophysiology, 49*, 1454–1463.

Makeig, S., Bell, A. J., Jung, T. P., & Sejnowski, T. J. (1996). Independent component analysis of electroencephalographic data. *Advances in Neural Information Processing Systems, 8*, 145–151.

Makeig, S., Jung, T. P., Bell, A. J., Ghahremani, D., & Sejnowski, T. J. (1997). Blind separation of auditory event-related brain responses into independent components. *Proceedings of the National Academy of Sciences of the United States of America, 94*(20), 10979–10984.

Makeig, S., Westerfield, M., Jung, T. P., Covington, J., Townsend, J., Sejnowski, T. J., & Courchesne, E. (1999). Functionally independent components of the late positive event-related potential during visual spatial attention. *The Journal of Neuroscience: The Official Journal of the Society for Neuroscience, 19*(7), 2665–2680.

Makeig, S., Westerfield, M., Townsend, J., Jung, T. P., Courchesne, E., & Sejnowski, T. J. (1999). Functionally independent components of early event-related potentials in a visual spatial attention task. *Philosophical Transactions of the Royal Society of London Series B, Biological Sciences, 354*(1387), 1135–1144. doi: 10.1098/rstb.1999.0469.

Marco-Pallares, J., Grau, C., & Ruffini, G. (2005). Combined ICA-LORETA analysis of mismatch negativity. *NeuroImage, 25*(2), 471–477. doi: 10.1016/j.neuroimage.2004.11.028.

Mennes, M., Wouters, H., Vanrumste, B., Lagae, L., & Stiers, P. (2010). Validation of ICA as a tool to remove eye movement artifacts from EEG/ERP. *Psychophysiology, 47*(6), 1142–1150. doi: 10.1111/j.1469-8986.2010.01015.x.

Minka, T. P. (2001). Automatic choice of dimensionality for PCA. *Advances in Neural Information Processing Systems, 15*, 604–604.

Näätänen, R., Kujala, T., Escera, C., Baldeweg, T., Kreegipuu, K., Carlson, C., & Ponton, C. (2012). The mismatch negativity (MMN) — A unique window to disturbed central auditory processing in ageing and different clinical conditions. *Clinical Neurophysiology: Official Journal of the International Federation of Clinical Neurophysiology, 123*, 424–458.

Näätänen, R., Kujala, T., Kreegipuu, K., Carlson, S., Escera, C., Baldeweg, T., & Ponton, C. (2011). The mismatch negativity: An index of cognitive decline in neuropsychiatric and neurological diseases and in ageing. *Brain: A Journal of Neurology, 134*(Pt 12), 3432–3450. doi: 10.1093/brain/awr064.

Onton, J., Westerfield, M., Townsend, J., & Makeig, S. (2006). Imaging human EEG dynamics using independent component analysis. *Neuroscience and Biobehavioral Reviews, 30*(6), 808–822. doi: 10.1016/j.neubiorev.2006.06.007.

Ortiz-Mantilla, S., Hämäläinen, J. A., & Benasich, A. A. (2012). Time course of ERP generators to syllables in infants: A source localization study using age-appropriate brain templates. *NeuroImage, 59*(4), 3275–3287. doi: 10.1016/j.neuroimage.2011.11.048.

Ortiz-Mantilla, S., Hämäläinen, J., Musacchia, G., & Benasich, A. (2013). Enhancement of gamma oscillations indicates preferential processing of native over foreign phonemic contrasts in infants. *The Journal of Neuroscience: The Official Journal of the Society for Neuroscience, 33*(48), 18746–18754.

Rissanen, J. (1978). Modeling by the shortest data description. *Automatica, 14*, 465–471.

Rossion, B. & Jacques, C. (2008). Does physical interstimulus variance account for early electrophysiological face sensitive responses in the human brain? Ten lessons on the N170. *NeuroImage, 39*(4), 1959–1979. doi: 10.1016/j.neuroimage.2007.10.011.

Schwarz, G. (1978). Estimating the dimension of a model. *Annals of Statistics, 6,* 461–464.

Seghouane, A. & Cichocki, A. (2007). Bayesian estimation of the number of principal components. *Signal Processing, 87,* 562–568.

Selen, Y. & Larsson, E. G. (2007). Empirical Bayes Linear Regression with Unknown Model Order. Paper presented at the 2007 *IEEE International Conference on Acoustics Speech and Signal Processing* (ICASSP 2007).

Shi, X. Z. (2011). *Blind Signal Processing: Theory and Practice.* Springer.

Stefanics, G., Csukly, G., Komlosi, S., Czobor, P., & Czigler, I. (2012). Processing of unattended facial emotions: A visual mismatch negativity study. *NeuroImage, 59*(3), 3042–3049. doi: 10.1016/j.neuroimage.2011.10.041.

Stoica, P. & Selen, Y. (2004). Model-order selection: A review of information criterion rules. *IEEE Signal Processing Magazine, 21*(4), 36–47.

Tan, P. N., Steinbach, M., & Kumar, V. (2005). *Introduction to Data Mining* (1st ed.). Addison-Wesley.

Ulfarsson, M. O. & Solo, V. (2008, 2008). Rank Selection in Noisy PCA with Sure and Random Matrix Theory. Paper presented at the 2008 *IEEE International Conference on Acoustics, Speech and Signal Processing* (ICASSP 2008).

Vakorin, V. A., Kovacevic, N., & McIntosh, A. R. (2010). Exploring transient transfer entropy based on a group-wise ICA decomposition of EEG data. *NeuroImage, 49*(2), 1593–1600. doi: 10.1016/j.neuroimage.2009.08.027.

Wax, M. & Kailath, T. (1985). Detection of signals by information theoretic criteria. *IEEE Transactions on Acoustics Speech and Signal Processing, 33,* 387–392.

Vigario, R. & Oja, E. (2008). BSS and ICA in neuroinformatics: From current practices to open challenges. *IEEE Reviews in Biomedical Engineering, 1,* 50–61.

Vigario, R., Sarela, J., Jousmaki, V., Hämäläinen, M., & Oja, E. (2000). Independent component approach to the analysis of EEG and MEG recordings. *IEEE Transactions on Bio-Medical Engineering, 47*(5), 589–593. doi: 10.1109/10.841330.

Zeman, P. M., Till, B. C., Livingston, N. J., Tanaka, J. W., & Driessen, P. F. (2007). Independent component analysis and clustering improve signal-to-noise ratio for statistical analysis of event-related potentials. *Clinical Neurophysiology: Official Journal of the International Federation of Clinical Neurophysiology, 118*(12), 2591–2604. doi: 10.1016/j.clinph.2007.09.00.

Chapter 4

Multi-Domain Feature of the ERP Extracted by NTF: New Approach for Group-Level Analysis of ERPs

In this chapter, we introduce a new group-level analysis approach for event-related potentials (ERPs). This approach is based on the multi-domain feature of the ERP extracted by nonnegative tensor factorization (NTF) from a high-order ERP tensor of the time-frequency representations (TFRs).

4.1 TFR of ERPs and High-Order Tensor

4.1.1 *TFR of ERPs: Evoked and induced brain activity*

The ERP measurements, including the peak latencies and amplitudes, are the most analyzed parameters in cognitive neuroscience (Luck, 2005). They reflect the ERP information in the time domain. To overcome the shortcoming of the ERP peak measurements, the ERP spectrum and the TFR of an ERP in the averaged and single-trial EEG data have been investigated (Cohen, 2014; Delorme & Makeig, 2004; Herrmann, Rach, Vosskuhl, & Struber, 2013). The TFR can be obtained from the absolute value of the wavelet transform (Daubechies, 1992) of the electroencephalography (EEG) data with a duration of one epoch.

4.1.1.1 *Difference in the TFR of an ERP between the evoked and induced brain activities*

In particular, the TFR of an ERP has two advantages. One advantage is that it can simultaneously exploit the temporal and spectral properties of the ERP. The other advantage is that it can reveal both the evoked and induced brain activities (David, Kilner, & Friston, 2006; Herrmann *et al.*, 2013; Tallon-Baudry, Bertrand, Delpuech, & Pernier, 1996).

Figure 4.1 shows one example (Bertrand & Tallon-Baudry, 2000). Figure 4.1(a) shows the EEG data of many single trials. Figure 4.1(b) shows the averaged EEG over the single trials in the time domain. Figure 4.1(c) shows the TFR of the averaged EEG. Figures 4.1(b) and (c) show that only the brain activity which is phase-locked to the stimulus among the single trials remains. Such brain activity is called evoked brain activity. Figure 4.1(d) shows the TFR of the EEG in each single trial, and Figure 4.1(e) shows the averaged TFR over the single trials. Figure 4.1(e) shows that the brain activity, which may be not phase-locked to the stimulus but elicited by the stimulus, remains. Such brain activity is called induced brain activity. Recently, studies on induced brain activity using TFR have become very popular (Axmacher *et al.*, 2010; Cavanagh, Cohen, & Allen, 2009; Debener, Ullsperger, Siegel, & Engel, 2006; Debener *et al.*, 2005; Stefanics *et al.*, 2007).

The function that analyzes induced brain activity by the TFR is currently provided in the commercial EEG data processing software Vision Analyzer (Brain Products GmbH) and open-source software EEGLAB (Delorme & Makeig, 2004). Moreover, in the ERP Boot Camp (a workshop on the ERP methods organized and led by Professor Steve Luck; http://erpinfo.org/the-erp-bootcamp), the TFR of an ERP is referred to as the TFR of induced brain activity in ERP experiments.

4.1.1.2 *TFR of an ERP used in this study: TFR of the averaged EEG*

The TFR of an ERP can refer to two different things, as shown in Figure 4.1. In ERP experiments that succeed in eliciting ERPs, the averaged TFR over single trials cannot always reveal the induced brain activity. This is because such brain activity largely depends on the experimental paradigm. Meanwhile, the TFR of the averaged EEG can

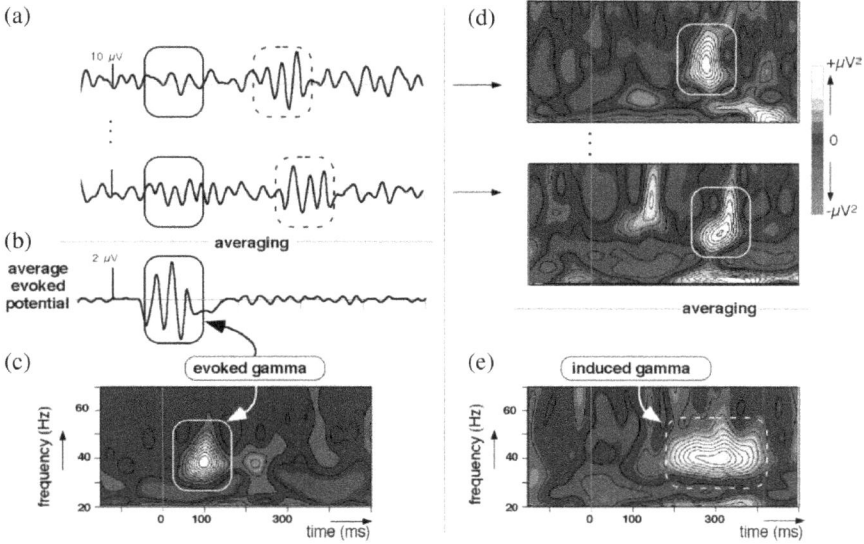

Figure 4.1 (a–e) TFR of ERPs: (c) evoked and (e) induced brain activity [adapted from Bertrand & Tallon-Baudry (2000)].

always exploit the temporal and spectral properties of the evoked brain activity.

Although both the TFR of the averaged EEG and the peak measurements of the ERP belong to the evoked brain activity, studying the TFR of the averaged EEG to analyze the ERP remains beneficial, in contrast to the peak measurement of the ERP. For example, we can observe how the brain activity simultaneously evolves in both time and frequency domains using the TFR (Herrmann *et al.*, 2013).

4.1.1.3 *ROI of the TFR of the ERP*

After the TFR of the ERP is derived, we need to determine the region of interest (ROI) to facilitate further statistical analysis such as the analysis of the peak measurements. For example, the rectangle in the TFR plane shown in Figure 4.1(c) is usually defined as the ROI. The rectangle depends on the time window and frequency range, which are often subjectively selected.

Therefore, objectively determining the ROI becomes a critical and significant research topic when TFR is used to analyze the ERPs. Chapter 3 discussed that the EEG data can be modeled using a linear transform model. If the mixture in the time-frequency domain can be separated, the component in the ROI can be extracted automatically. In this chapter, we show that the NTF is an excellent tool for this purpose.

4.1.2 High-order ERP tensor

A multi-way data array is called a tensor. In ERP experiments, many tensors exist.

4.1.2.1 ERP waveform tensors

The EEG data in ERP experiments include many modes, namely, time, space, trial, stimulus, and participant. Therefore, single-trial EEG data can assemble a five-way array, i.e., fifth-order tensor. The averaged EEG data over single trials can compose a fourth-order tensor. Moreover, if the stimulus and participant modes are merged, a third-order tensor can be produced.

Usually, different modes are stacked or concatenated to produce a two-way array. For example, different single trials, different subjects, or different stimuli can be concatenated for a group-level ICA (Delorme & Makeig, 2004; Eichele, Rachakonda, Brakedal, Eikeland, & Calhoun, 2011; Kovacevic & McIntosh, 2007). This process indicates that the inherent high-order structures of ERP data in ERP experiments are seldom exploited (Vanderperren *et al.*, 2013).

4.1.2.2 ERP tensors of TFRs of averaged EEG data

Given the EEG data of a single trial or the averaged EEG data of one stimulus and one participant in an ERP experiment, two modes naturally exist, namely, time and space. If the EEG data at each channel are transformed into the time-frequency domain, the new data include three modes: time, frequency, and space. Figure 4.2 shows an example of the TFRs of the EEG data in multiple channels (Zhao *et al.*, 2011).

As mentioned in the previous section, the averaged EEG data in ERP experiments may include four modes: time, space, stimulus, and participant. After the averaged EEG data are transformed into the time-frequency domain, a fifth-order tensor that includes the TFR of the averaged EEG

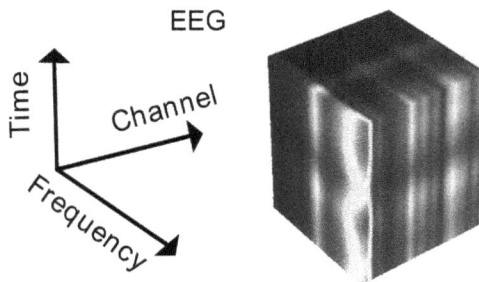

Figure 4.2 Example of a third-order tensor: time-frequency representation of the EEG data in multiple channels [adapted from Zhao *et al.* (2011)].

data is produced with five modes: time, frequency, space, stimulus, and participant. If the stimulus and participant modes are merged, a fourth-order tensor is generated. If the stimulus, participant, and space are stacked together, a third-order tensor is composed.

When the EEG data are represented by a matrix, matrix decomposition methods such as the principal component analysis (PCA) and independent component analysis (ICA) can be applied to process the EEG data. Similarly, when the EEG data are represented by a tensor, tensor decomposition methods (Acar & Yener, 2009; Cichocki *et al.*, 2014; Cichocki, Zdunek, Phan & Amari, 2009; Kolda & Bader, 2009; Kroonenberg, 2008; Smilde, Bro & Geladi, 2004) can be used to extract the components of interest in the different modes. In the next section, we introduce the tensor decomposition method to analyze the ERP data.

4.2 Introduction of the Tensor Decomposition

4.2.1 *Brief history*

Tensor decomposition based on a canonical polyadic (CP) model was studied way back in 1927 (Hitchcock, 1927). For a very long time, little progress has been made in tensor decomposition. In 1966, tensor decomposition based on the Tucker model was proposed (Tucker, 1966). Because these two studies belong to the field of mathematics, they did not attract much attention from other disciplines. In 1970, two independent but similar studies (Carroll & Chang, 1970; Harshman, 1970) in the field of psychometrics were published. Thereafter, an increasing number of researchers in various fields have started working on the theory and application of tensor decomposition. One of the most important applications for tensor decomposition is chemometrics (Bro, 1998; Kroonenberg, 2008; Smilde *et al.*, 2004). In 2009, an important review paper for tensor decomposition (Kolda & Bader, 2009) was published in the journal *SIAM Review*. By March 2014, the paper has been cited over 400 times in the Web of Knowledge.

In the field of signal processing, tensor decomposition has also drawn extensive attention (Cichocki *et al.*, 2014). In particular, tensor decomposition has become an important tool in analyzing large-scale brain data (Beckmann & Smith, 2005; Cichocki, 2013; Morup, Hansen, & Arnfred, 2007) in the field of brain science.

For a very long time, tensor decomposition has been known as parallel factor analysis (PARAFAC) (Harshman, 1970). Indeed, PARAFAC and CP decomposition (CPD) (Hitchcock, 1927) are equivalent. Therefore, we use CPD instead of PARAFAC hereinafter in this book.

4.2.2 *Basis for tensor decomposition*

To avoid complicated mathematics in the tensor decomposition algorithms, we only introduce the basic products of tensor decomposition.

4.2.2.1 *Inner and outer products*

The inner and outer products are very fundamental in tensor decomposition. Given two column vectors $\mathbf{a} = [a_1, a_2, a_3]^T$ and $\mathbf{b} = [b_1, b_2, b_3]^T$, their inner product is

$$x = \mathbf{a}^T \cdot \mathbf{b} = a_1 \cdot b_1 + a_2 \cdot b_2 + a_3 \cdot b_3,$$

and their outer product is

$$\mathbf{X} = \mathbf{a} \circ \mathbf{b} = \begin{bmatrix} a_1 \cdot b_1 & a_1 \cdot b_2 & a_1 \cdot b_3 \\ a_2 \cdot b_1 & a_2 \cdot b_2 & a_2 \cdot b_3 \\ a_3 \cdot b_1 & a_3 \cdot b_2 & a_3 \cdot b_3 \end{bmatrix} = \mathbf{a} \cdot \mathbf{b}^T, \quad x_{ij} = a_i \cdot b_j,$$

where the symbol "∘" denotes the outer product of the vectors.

4.2.2.2 *Outer product of multiple vectors*

Given three vectors $\mathbf{a} \in \Re^{I \times 1}$, $\mathbf{b} \in \Re^{J \times 1}$, and $\mathbf{c} \in \Re^{K \times 1}$, their outer product yields a third-order rank-one tensor

$$\underline{\mathbf{X}} = \mathbf{a} \circ \mathbf{b} \circ \mathbf{c} \in \Re^{I \times J \times K},$$

where $x_{ijk} = a_i b_j c_k$, $i = 1, \ldots, I$, $j = 1, \ldots, J$, and $k = 1, \ldots, K$. This tensor is called a rank-one tensor.

4.2.2.3 *Mode-n tensor matrix product*

The mode-n product $\underline{\mathbf{X}} = \underline{\mathbf{G}} \times_n \mathbf{A}$ of tensor $\underline{\mathbf{G}} \in \Re^{J_1 \times J_2 \times \cdots \times J_N}$ and matrix $\mathbf{A} \in \mathbb{R}^{I_n \times J_n}$ is tensor $\underline{\mathbf{X}} \in \underline{\Re}^{J_1 \times J_2 \times \cdots \times J_{n-1} \times I_n \times J_{n+1} \times \cdots \times J_N}$ with the following elements:

$$x_{j_1 j_2 \cdots j_{n-1} i_n j_{n+1} \cdots j_N} = \sum_{j_n=1}^{J_n} g_{j_1 j_2 \cdots j_N} a_{i_n, j_n}.$$

4.2.3 *CPD model*

4.2.3.1 *Simple illustration of the CPD*

Given a third-order tensor, a two-component CPD is shown in Figure 4.3 (Bro, 1998).

$$\underline{\mathbf{X}} \approx \mathbf{a}_1 \circ \mathbf{b}_1 \circ \mathbf{c}_1 + \mathbf{a}_2 \circ \mathbf{b}_2 \circ \mathbf{c}_2 = \underline{\mathbf{X}}_1 + \underline{\mathbf{X}}_2. \tag{4-1}$$

As an example, a third-order tensor is shown in Figure 4.2. After the two-component CPD is applied on the tensor, two temporal, two spectral, and two spatial components are extracted, as shown in Figure 4.3. In this application, the first temporal component $\mathbf{a}_1$, the first spectral component $\mathbf{b}_1$, and the first spatial component $\mathbf{c}_1$ are associated with one another, and their outer product produces rank-one tensor $\underline{\mathbf{X}}_1$. The second components

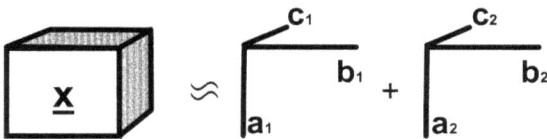

Figure 4.3   Two-component CPD of a third-order tensor [adapted from Bro (1998)].

in the time, frequency, and space modes are associated with one another, and their outer product generates rank-one tensor $\underline{\mathbf{X}}_2$. The sum of rank-one tensors $\underline{\mathbf{X}}_1$ and $\underline{\mathbf{X}}_2$ approximates original tensor $\underline{\mathbf{X}}$.

4.2.3.2 *General definition of CPD*

Generally, for a given Nth-order tensor $\underline{\mathbf{X}} \in \mathfrak{R}^{I_1 \times I_2 \times \cdots \times I_N}$, the CPD is defined as

$$\underline{\mathbf{X}} = \sum_{r=1}^{R} \mathbf{u}_r^{(1)} \circ \mathbf{u}_r^{(2)} \circ \cdots \circ \mathbf{u}_r^{(N)} + \underline{\mathbf{E}} = \sum_{r=1}^{R} \underline{\mathbf{X}}_r + \underline{\mathbf{E}} = \underline{\hat{\mathbf{X}}} + \underline{\mathbf{E}}, \quad (4\text{-}2)$$

where $\underline{\mathbf{X}}_r = \mathbf{u}_r^{(1)} \circ \mathbf{u}_r^{(2)} \circ \cdots \circ \mathbf{u}_r^{(N)}$, $r = 1, 2, \ldots, R$; $\underline{\hat{\mathbf{X}}}$ approximates tensor $\underline{\mathbf{X}}$, $\underline{\mathbf{E}} \in \mathfrak{R}^{I_1 \times I_2 \times \cdots \times I_N}$; and $\|\mathbf{u}_r^{(n)}\|_2 = 1$, for $n = 1, 2, \ldots, N - 1$.

Therefore, CPD is the sum of the R rank-one tensors plus the error tensor. Rank-one tensor #r is the outer product of N components from N component matrices, and each component is the component #r among the R components contained in each component matrix.

In the tensor-matrix product form, Eq. (4-2) transforms into

$$\underline{\mathbf{X}} = \underline{\mathbf{I}} \times_1 \mathbf{U}^{(1)} \times_2 \mathbf{U}^{(2)} \times_3 \cdots \times_N \mathbf{U}^{(N)} + \underline{\mathbf{E}} = \underline{\hat{\mathbf{X}}} + \underline{\mathbf{E}}, \quad (4\text{-}3)$$

where $\underline{\mathbf{I}}$ is an identity tensor, which is a diagonal tensor with a diagonal entry of one. $\mathbf{U}^{(n)} = [\mathbf{u}_1^{(n)}, \mathbf{u}_2^{(n)}, \ldots, \mathbf{u}_R^{(n)}] \in \mathfrak{R}^{I_n \times R}$ denotes a component matrix for model #n, and $n = 1, 2, \ldots, N$.

4.2.3.3 *Uniqueness analysis of CPD*

Furthermore, when the CPD is subjected to permutation and variance indeterminacies, a theoretical unique CPD for Eq. (4-2) exists without requiring any additional assumptions (Cichocki *et al.*, 2014; Kolda & Bader, 2009). This condition is the outstanding advantage of tensor decomposition based on the CP model.

The uniqueness of the CPD on a high-order tensor can be examined using a variant of the Kruskal's theorem (Kruskal, 1977; Sidiropoulos & Bro, 2000) as follows:

$$\sum_{n=1}^{N} r_{\mathbf{U}^{(n)}} \geq 2R + N - 1,$$

where $r_{\mathbf{U}^{(n)}}$ is the rank of component matrix $\mathbf{U}^{(n)}$ in Eq. (4-3), R is the number of extracted components from each mode, and N is the number of modes for a given tensor.

We should note that $\mathbf{U}^{(n)}$ may not be a full-rank matrix because some columns of the component matrix in Eq. (4-3) can be very much correlated both in theory and in practice.

4.2.3.4 *Difference between matrix decomposition and CPD*

If $N = 2$, Eq. (4-2) degenerates into a matrix decomposition as

$$\mathbf{X} = \sum_{r=1}^{R} \mathbf{u}_r^{(1)} \circ \mathbf{u}_r^{(2)} + \mathbf{E} = \mathbf{X} + \mathbf{E}. \qquad (4\text{-}4)$$

Indeed, Eq. (4-4) is the model for blind source separation (BSS) (Cichocki & Amari, 2003; Comon, 1994; Comon & Jutten, 2010; Hyvarinen, Karhunen, & Oja, 2001). Therefore, we can state that Eq. (4-4) is a blind separation of a mixture with two modes, and Eq. (4-2) is a blind separation of a mixture with N modes (Cichocki *et al.*, 2009, 2014).

Without making additional assumptions, no unique matrix decomposition is available for Eq. (4-4). This is the main difference between the matrix decomposition and CPD.

When the assumptions required by ICA are met, the ICA decomposition in Eq. (4-4) can be unique from the matrix decomposition subject to the permutation and variance indeterminacies (Cichocki & Amari, 2003; Comon, 1994; Comon & Jutten, 2010; Hyvarinen *et al.*, 2001).

4.2.4 *Tucker decomposition model*

For a given Nth-order tensor $\underline{\mathbf{X}} \in \Re^{I_1 \times I_2 \times \cdots \times I_N}$, the Tucker decomposition is expressed as follows:

$$\underline{\mathbf{X}} = \sum_{r_1=1}^{R_1} \sum_{r_2=1}^{R_2} \cdots \sum_{r_N=1}^{R_N} g_{r_1 r_2 \cdots r_N} \mathbf{a}_{r_1}^{(1)} \circ \mathbf{a}_{r_2}^{(2)} \circ \cdots \circ \mathbf{a}_{r_N}^{(N)} + \underline{\mathbf{E}}$$

$$= \sum_{r_1=1}^{R_1} \sum_{r_2=1}^{R_2} \cdots \sum_{r_N=1}^{R_N} g_{r_1 r_2 \cdots r_N} \underline{\mathbf{X}}_{r_1 r_2 \cdots r_N} + \underline{\mathbf{E}}, \qquad (4\text{-}5)$$

where rank-one tensor $\underline{\mathbf{X}}_{r_1 r_2 \cdots r_N} = \mathbf{a}_{r_1}^{(1)} \circ \mathbf{a}_{r_2}^{(2)} \circ \cdots \circ \mathbf{a}_{r_N}^{(N)}$, $I_n \geq R_n$, and $g_{r_1 r_2 \cdots r_N}$ composes the core tensor $\underline{\mathbf{G}} \in \mathfrak{R}^{R_1 \times R_2 \times \cdots \times R_N}$. To avoid unnecessary confusion, we denote the component in the Tucker decomposition by $\mathbf{a}$ instead of $\mathbf{u}$ in the CPD.

Therefore, the Tucker decomposition is the sum of the $R_1 \times R_2 \times \cdots \times R_N$ scaled rank-one tensors plus the error tensor. Each rank-one tensor is the outer product of N components from N component matrices, and each component is from the component matrix among the N matrices.

In the tensor-matrix form, Eq. (4-5) is transformed into

$$\underline{\mathbf{X}} = \underline{\mathbf{G}} \times_1 \mathbf{A}^{(1)} \times_2 \mathbf{A}^{(2)} \times_3 \cdots \times_N \mathbf{A}^{(N)} + \underline{\mathbf{E}} = \hat{\underline{\mathbf{X}}} + \underline{\mathbf{E}}, \qquad (4\text{-}6)$$

where $\mathbf{A}^{(n)} = [\mathbf{a}_1^{(n)}, \mathbf{a}_2^{(n)}, \ldots, \mathbf{a}_{R_n}^{(n)}] \in \mathfrak{R}^{I_n \times R_n}$ $(n = 1, 2, \ldots, N)$ denotes the component matrix. To avoid confusion, we denote the component matrix in the Tucker decomposition by $\mathbf{A}$ instead of $\mathbf{U}$ in the CPD.

In theory, the Tucker decomposition does not possess unique solutions even though it is subjected to the permutation and variance indeterminacies (Cichocki *et al.*, 2014; Kolda & Bader, 2009). In practice, when additional assumptions are introduced on the different modes, the Tucker decomposition can be relatively unique (Zhou & Cichocki, 2012).

4.2.5 *Difference between the CPD and Tucker decomposition models*

In terms of the tensor decomposition models, four main differences exist between the CPD and Tucker decomposition.

(1) In the CPD, the number of components in the different modes remains invariant. However, in the Tucker decomposition, the number of components in the different modes can be different.

(2) Both the CPD and Tucker decomposition are derived in terms of the sum of rank-one tensors, and each rank-one tensor is the outer product of N components from N component matrices with N modes. However, the requirements of the N components used to compose the rank-one tensor are different. In the CPD, each of the N components that produce the rank-one tensor must be the component #r of each component matrix among the N component matrices of N modes. In the Tucker decomposition, each component comes from each component matrix, and no limitation is imposed on the order of the chosen component in

the component matrix. In other words, the components of the different component matrices in the CPD are associated with one another only when the components have the same index among the R indexes. This condition means that in Eq. (4-2), $\mathbf{u}_r^{(n_1)}$ and $\mathbf{u}_r^{(n_2)}$ are associated with each other ($n_1 \in [1, N]$ and $n_2 \in [1, N]$); however, $\mathbf{u}_{r_1}^{(n_1)}$ and $\mathbf{u}_{r_2}^{(n_2)}$ are not associated with each other when $r_1 \neq r_2$ ($r_1 \in [1, R]$, $r_2 \in [1, R]$) irrespective if n_1 and n_2 are equal or not. For example, in Figure 4.3, the first temporal component $\mathbf{a}_1$, first spectral component $\mathbf{b}_1$, and first spatial component $\mathbf{c}_1$ are associated with one another, but any of them is not associated with $\mathbf{a}_2$, $\mathbf{b}_2$, or $\mathbf{c}_2$. In the Tucker decomposition, any component from the different component matrices can be associated with one another.

(3) The core tensor in the CPD is the identity tensor, but that in the Tucker decomposition is not the identity tensor.

(4) In theory, when the tensor decomposition is subjected to the permutation and variance indeterminacies, the CPD can be unique; however, the Tucker decomposition cannot be unique when no additional assumptions are introduced.

Because of these four differences, the Tucker decomposition can more possibly factorize a tensor than the CPD (Cichocki *et al.*, 2014; Kolda & Bader, 2009).

4.2.6 *Fit of a tensor decomposition model*

Regardless of whether the CPD or Tucker decomposition is used, the sum of the rank-one tensors approximates the factorized tensor. Therefore, the sum simply explains parts of the variance in the factorized tensor. Then, a parameter called "fit" is defined to determine the degree of variance.

$$\text{fit} = 1 - \frac{\|\mathbf{X} - \hat{\mathbf{X}}\|_F}{\|\mathbf{X}\|_F}, \tag{4-7}$$

where $\hat{\mathbf{X}} = \sum_{r=1}^{R} \mathbf{X}_r$ and $\mathbf{X}_r$ for the CPD are defined in Eq. (4-2) and $\hat{\mathbf{X}} = \sum_{r_1=1}^{R_1} \sum_{r_2=1}^{R_2} \cdots \sum_{r_N=1}^{R_N} g_{r_1 r_2 \cdots r_N} \underline{\mathbf{X}}_{r_1 r_2 \cdots r_N}$, and $\underline{\mathbf{X}}_{r_1 r_2 \cdots r_N}$ for the Tucker decomposition are defined in Eq. (4-5). $\| \cdot \|_F$ is the Frobenius norm of the tensor (Cichocki *et al.*, 2009). Norm-1 (absolute value) is also often used to calculate the fit.

Obviously, fit is not more than one. With the increase in the number of components, the fit also increases. However, a larger fit does not mean a better tensor decomposition. Fit is largely affected by the level of noise in a tensor and the CPD and Tucker decomposition models.

4.2.7 *Classic algorithms of the CPD and Tucker decomposition*

Most algorithms for tensor decomposition minimize the squared Euclidean distance (Frobenius norm), which is regarded as a cost function (Acar & Yener, 2009; Bro, 1998; Cichocki *et al.*, 2009, 2014; Kolda & Bader, 2009; Kroonenberg, 2008; Smilde *et al.*, 2004).

For the CPD, the cost function is given by

$$D(\underline{\mathbf{X}}|\hat{\underline{\mathbf{X}}}) = \frac{1}{2}\|\underline{\mathbf{X}} - \underline{\mathbf{I}} \times_1 \mathbf{U}^{(1)} \times_2 \mathbf{U}^{(2)} \times_3 \cdots \times_N \mathbf{U}^{(N)}\|_F^2. \qquad (4\text{-}8)$$

For the Tucker decomposition, the cost function is

$$D(\underline{\mathbf{X}}|\underline{\mathbf{G}}, \{\mathbf{A}\}) = \frac{1}{2}\|\underline{\mathbf{X}} - \underline{\mathbf{G}} \times_1 \mathbf{A}^{(1)} \times_2 \mathbf{A}^{(2)} \times_3 \cdots \times_N \mathbf{A}^{(N)}\|_F^2. \qquad (4\text{-}9)$$

To minimize the cost functions for the CPD and Tucker decomposition, alternating least square (ALS) is one of the fundamental and classic optimization approaches to derive the tensor decomposition algorithms (Acar & Yener, 2009; Bro, 1998; Cichocki *et al.*, 2009, 2014; Kolda & Bader, 2009; Kroonenberg, 2008; Smilde *et al.*, 2004).

In practice, all component matrices of the CPD are initialized following an initialization method. For the Tucker decomposition, the core tensor is also initialized. The commonly used methods include randomization, fiber, and singular value decomposition (Cichocki *et al.*, 2009). After the parameters are initialized and the number of extracted component by the CPD is selected, the ALS first fixes all the component matrices except one and then calculates the derivative of the cost function with respect to the unfixed component matrix. The derivative calculation is sequentially alternated over each component matrix in each mode. After the first alternating iteration on all modes, the fit is calculated. If the fit is smaller than the predefined threshold, the iteration is stopped. Otherwise, the second iteration is started, and all modes are sequentially alternated to calculate the derivative. The iteration does not stop until some predefined criteria are met. For the Tucker decomposition, both the core tensor and the component matrices are included in the alternating derivative calculation.

The ALS approach is based on the derivative of the cost function with respect to each component matrix. Indeed, the hierarchical ALS (HALS) algorithm is more efficient, and it is based on the derivative of the cost function with respect to each column (i.e., each component) of each component matrix (Cichocki, Zdunek, & Amari, 2007).

Furthermore, when the mode size of a tensor is very large, redundant information is present in that mode. Therefore, the low-rank approximation (LRA) method (Zhou, Cichocki, & Xie, 2012) can be applied to simultaneously reduce the mode and the tensor sizes, which can dramatically improve the computing efficiency (Cong *et al.*, 2014; Zhou *et al.*, 2012).

4.2.8 *NTF*

Section 4.1 stated that the TFR value of a signal is nonnegative. In this book, we define a tensor and a matrix where both have all nonnegative elements as a nonnegative tensor and a nonnegative matrix, respectively.

When tensor decomposition is used to factorize a nonnegative tensor, nonnegative constraints are often applied. This process means that each component in Eqs. (4-2) and (4-3) of the CPD and each component in Eqs. (4-5) and (4-6) in the Tucker decomposition are forced to be nonnegative after each iteration of the tensor decomposition algorithm (please see Section 4.2.7).

To conform with historical convention, the tensor decomposition with nonnegative constraints is denoted as NTF (Kolda & Bader, 2009). NTF also includes two basic models. The CPD with nonnegative constraints is called nonnegative CPD (NCPD) (Cong, Phan, *et al.*, 2013; Cong *et al.*, 2014), and the Tucker decomposition with nonnegative constraints is called nonnegative Tucker decomposition (NTD) (Phan & Cichocki, 2011).

4.2.9 *Why is a nonnegative ERP tensor of the TFR used instead of an ERP tensor of a waveform?*

The data of various ERP tensors introduced in Section 4.1.2 have some underlying properties, e.g., independence among sources, sparsity of topography, nonnegativity of the TFR, etc. Among these properties, only the nonnegativity of the TFR is certainly objective.

For the matrix decomposition, nonnegative matrix factorization (NMF) (Lee & Seung, 1999) has been shown to be superior over many other matrix decomposition methods of nonnegative matrices (Cichocki *et al.*, 2009), such as the PCA and BSS.

Recently, CPD on the ERP tensor of the averaged EEG data waveforms has been shown not to produce components that are as satisfactory as the NCPD on the ERP tensor of the TFRs of the averaged EEG data (Cong *et al.*, 2014). The CPD with inappropriate constraints did not well separate the mixtures represented by the ERP tensor of the waveforms (Cong *et al.*, 2014). The NCPD extracted more reasonable ERP components from the nonnegative TFR of the ERP data (Cong *et al.*, 2014). We believe the key reason is that the ERP tensor of the TFRs is nonnegative, and it is natural and objective to add the nonnegative constraint in the tensor decomposition.

Furthermore, the TFR of the ERP component is very sparse. Examining the sparse property is easy by referring to the TFRs shown in Figures 4.1 and 4.2. The implicit addition of the sparse constraints enhances the decomposition of the mixture into underlying components in two modes by the ICA (Daubechies *et al.*, 2009). Consequently, forcing the nonnegative constraints implicitly adds the sparse constraint to the NTF, which helps in the separation of the mixtures represented by the nonnegative tensor.

4.3 Multi-Domain Feature of ERP

4.3.1 *Conventional features of an ERP (averaged EEG) versus features of spontaneous and single-trial EEGs*

4.3.1.1 *Conventional features of an ERP (averaged EEG)*

The statistical test of the ERP measurements is a necessary part in ERP studies. Conventional measurements include the peak amplitude and latency in the time domain (Luck, 2005), power of the event-related oscillation in the time or frequency domain (Basar, 2004; Basar, Schurmann, Demiralp, Basar-Eroglu, & Ademoglu, 2001; Gorsev & Basar, 2010; Ramos-Loyo, Gonzalez-Garrido, Sanchez-Loyo, Medina, & Basar-Eroglu, 2009; Yener,

Guntekin, Oniz & Basar, 2007), and ROI value in the time-frequency domain (Bishop & Hardiman, 2010; Delorme & Makeig, 2004; Fuentemilla, Marco-Pallares, Munte & Grau, 2008; Herrmann *et al.*, 2013; Stefanics *et al.*, 2007).

We should note that after any of these measurements are performed on each channel, the measurement topography is available. This means that the ERP properties in the time, or/and the frequency and in spatial domains are sequentially exploited.

Such ERP measurements can be represented by the ERP features in the fields of machine learning and pattern recognition. We use these features hereafter.

4.3.1.2 *Features of spontaneous and single-trial EEGs for pattern recognition*

The feature extraction of spontaneous EEG for clinical diagnosis of neurological disorders (Adeli & Ghosh-Dastidar, 2010) and for single-trial EEG for brain–computer interface (BCI) (Tan & Nijholt, 2010) has been very well developed. After the features are extracted, they are analyzed using pattern recognition methods (Bishop, 2006) to draw some conclusions.

For the spontaneous EEG, the features are mainly based on the temporal, spectral, and time-frequency properties and the complexity of the brain dynamics (Adeli & Ghosh-Dastidar, 2010). Some features are obtained by complicated mathematical transforms, e.g., complexity of the brain dynamics. For the single-trial EEG for BCI, the features are mainly obtained in terms of the EEG temporal, spectral, and spatial properties.

4.3.1.3 *Difference between the conventional features of an ERP for cognitive neuroscience and the features of spontaneous and single-trial EEGs for pattern recognition*

In ERP studies, statistical analysis using two or multiple factors is often applied on the ERP feature to determine the experimental effects (Luck, 2005). The factors often include the stimulus type (e.g., "standard" versus "deviant" in the oddball paradigm), hemisphere ("left" versus "right"), group ("control" versus "clinical"), etc. The important characteristic is that the ERP feature for the statistical tests should be cognitive, which means that the feature should straightforwardly demonstrate the ERP properties in the time, frequency, time-frequency, or spatial domain.

In the analysis of the spontaneous or single-trial EEGs in BCI, all feature types mentioned earlier are usually grouped, and some of them are finally selected for pattern recognition. Sometimes, all features are transformed to produce more discriminative features for pattern recognition. In such studies, which features are actually used do not matter as long as the pattern recognition is successful.

The pattern recognition methods can be divided into two groups, namely, unsupervised and supervised approaches. Figure 3.22 shows the clustering, which belongs to the unsupervised approach that does not use the cluster labels during the clustering. However, the supervised pattern recognition approach is often used in clinical diagnosis of neurological disorders and BCI. This approach means that the difference among the groups or tasks is already known, and the labels of the different groups or tasks are used during training step in the pattern recognition. In other words, the supervised pattern recognition methods are expressed in terms of *a priori* knowledge, i.e., the known group or task difference.

Therefore, the application of the features of the spontaneous and single-trial EEGs in BCI is very different from that of the conventional features of the ERPs. The purpose of the statistical analysis [e.g., analysis of variance (ANOVA)] of the conventional ERP features is to examine and show the group or task difference. In such statistical analysis, the group or task labels are not used at all.

Because of these differences, the spontaneous and single-trial EEG features in BCI cannot be straightforwardly applied for analyzing ERPs for the cognitive neuroscience.

4.3.2 *Brief review of the EEG data analysis by tensor decomposition*

The tensor decomposition based on the CP model has been applied to analyze the ERPs under one condition with one subject (Achim & Bouchard, 1997; Field & Graupe, 1991; Mocks, 1988a,b; Wang, Begleiter, & Porjesz, 2000). After the year 2000, increasing number of studies have used tensor decomposition to analyze the TFRs of EEGs and single-trial EEG (Acar, Aykut-Bingol, Bingol, Bro, & Yener, 2007; Acar, Bingol, & Bingol, 2006;

Acar, Bingol, Bingol, Bro, & Yener, 2007; Acar & Yener, 2009; Cichocki *et al.*, 2008; Cong, Phan, Zhao, Nandi, *et al.*, 2012; De Vos, De Lathauwer, Vanrumste, Van Huffel, & Van Paesschen, 2007; De Vos, Vergult, *et al.*, 2007; Deburchgraeve *et al.*, 2009; Eliseyev & Aksenova, 2013; Eliseyev *et al.*, 2012; Miwakeichi *et al.*, 2004; Morup, Hansen, Herrmann, Parnas, & Arnfred, 2006; Phan & Cichocki, 2010, 2011; Vanderperren *et al.*, 2013). These studies can be divided into two categories. One category indicates that a third-order ERP tensor of the waveforms or TFRs can be decomposed into a predefined number of components with different modes. The other category demonstrates that the new ERP features can be extracted by tensor decomposition, and these features can be used for pattern recognition.

Until 2007, the analysis of ERPs by tensor decomposition has not been like that of ERP's peak measurements for the cognitive neuroscience (Cong, Phan, Astikainen, *et al.*, 2012; Cong, Phan, *et al.*, 2013; Cong, Phan, Zhao, Huttunen-Scott, *et al.*, 2012; Cong *et al.*, 2014; Morup *et al.*, 2007). In these studies, the new ERP features were extracted by tensor decomposition from the ERP tensor of the TFRs. The effects of the ERP experiments were revealed by statistically analyzing the new features. In the next section, we introduce the extraction methods of the new cognitive features by the NTF and the analysis by statistical tests in cognitive neuroscience.

4.3.3 *Multi-domain feature of ERPs extracted by NCPD from the fourth-order ERP tensor of TFRs*

4.3.3.1 *Feature extraction*

When a fourth-order ERP tensor of the TFRs includes the time, frequency, space, and feature modes (the feature mode can include "participant" and "stimulus"), it can be decomposed into four component matrices of the four modes by NCPD as follows:

$$\underline{X} = \underline{I} \times_1 U^{(t)} \times_2 U^{(s)} \times_3 U^{(c)} \times_4 F + \underline{E}$$

$$= \sum_{r=1}^{R} \mathbf{u}_r^{(t)} \circ \mathbf{u}_r^{(s)} \circ \mathbf{u}_r^{(c)} \circ \mathbf{f}_r + \underline{E}, \qquad (4\text{-}10)$$

where $U^{(t)} = [\mathbf{u}_1^{(t)}, \mathbf{u}_2^{(t)}, \ldots, \mathbf{u}_R^{(t)}] \in \Re^{I_t \times R}$ denotes the temporal component matrix, $U^{(s)} = [\mathbf{u}_1^{(s)}, \mathbf{u}_2^{(s)}, \ldots, \mathbf{u}_R^{(s)}] \in \Re^{I_s \times R}$ represents the spectral

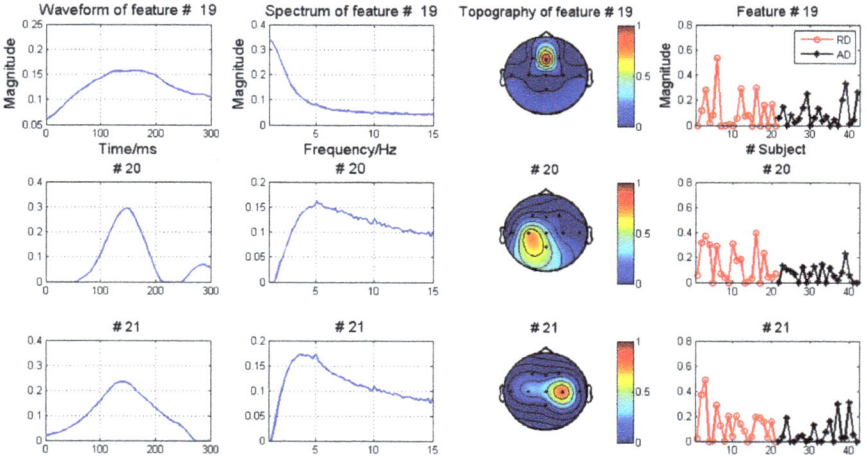

Figure 4.4 Example of NCPD on a fourth-order ERP tensor of the TFRs. The sizes of the tensor are 60 (temporal samples) × 71 (frequency bins) × 9 (channels) × 42 (the subjects are composed of two groups with 21 children per group). $R = 36$ for the NCPD, i.e., 36 components are extracted from each mode. Three of the 36 components are shown in each mode. The order of the components and the variance of a component in the NCPD are not determined. RD: reading disability. AD: attention deficit [adapted from Cong, Phan, Zhao, Huttunen-Scott, *et al.* (2012)].

component matrix, $\mathbf{U}^{(c)} = [\mathbf{u}_1^{(c)}, \mathbf{u}_2^{(c)}, \ldots, \mathbf{u}_R^{(c)}] \in \Re^{I_c \times R}$ is the channel/spatial component matrix, and $\mathbf{F} = [\mathbf{f}_1, \mathbf{f}_2, \ldots, \mathbf{f}_R] \in \Re^{I \times R}$ represents the multi-domain feature component matrix.

Figure 4.4 shows an example of the NCPD on a fourth-order ERP tensor of the TFRs that includes the time, frequency, space, and feature modes (Cong, Phan, Zhao, Huttunen-Scott, *et al.*, 2012). The ERP is elicited from the mismatch negativity (MMN) by the oddball paradigm shown in Figure A.4. For this example, $R = 36$ in Eq. (4-10). Then, the NCPD on the fourth-order tensor is expressed as

$$\underline{\mathbf{X}} = \mathbf{u}_1^{(t)} \circ \mathbf{u}_1^{(s)} \circ \mathbf{u}_1^{(c)} \circ \mathbf{f}_1 + \cdots + \mathbf{u}_{19}^{(t)} \circ \mathbf{u}_{19}^{(s)} \circ \mathbf{u}_{19}^{(c)} \circ \mathbf{f}_{19}$$
$$+ \mathbf{u}_{20}^{(t)} \circ \mathbf{u}_{20}^{(s)} \circ \mathbf{u}_{20}^{(c)} \circ \mathbf{f}_{20} + \mathbf{u}_{21}^{(t)} \circ \mathbf{u}_{21}^{(s)} \circ \mathbf{u}_{21}^{(c)} \circ \mathbf{f}_{21}$$
$$+ \cdots + \mathbf{u}_{36}^{(t)} \circ \mathbf{u}_{36}^{(s)} \circ \mathbf{u}_{36}^{(c)} \circ \mathbf{f}_{36} + \underline{\mathbf{E}}.$$

Components #19, #20, and #21 in each of the four modes are shown in Figure 4.4. Reckoned from the left to the right side, the first column in

Figure 4.4 shows three temporal components (#19–#21), which are the three columns of temporal component matrix $\mathbf{U}^{(t)}$; the second column describes the three spectral components (#19–#21), which are the three columns of spectral component matrix $\mathbf{U}^{(s)}$; the third column presents the three spatial components (i.e., topographies) (#19–#21), which are the three columns of spatial component matrix $\mathbf{U}^{(c)}$; and the last column shows the three multi-domain feature components (#19–#21), which are the three columns (#19–#21) of feature component matrix $\mathbf{F}$.

Obviously, the temporal, spectral, and spatial component matrices do not contain any information on the individual subjects, and they are common to all features. Variability among individual subjects exists in each feature component, which is a column of the feature component matrix. This is a characteristic of the multi-domain feature extraction of ERP when NCPD is applied on the fourth-order ERP tensor of the TFR that includes the time, frequency, space, and feature modes.

4.3.3.2 *Feature selection*

After the matrix decomposition such as ICA on the EEG, we need to choose the components of interest for further data processing. This process should also be done in the tensor decomposition. When ICA extracts the ERP component of a subject, the temporal and spatial properties of the ERP are used (please see Section 3.7.5). When NCPD is applied on the fourth-order ERP tensor of the TFRs, the temporal, spectral, and spatial components are extracted, in addition to the multi-domain features. Therefore, the ERP temporal, spectral, and spatial properties can be used to select its desired multi-domain feature, meaning that provided the temporal, spectral, and spatial components meet the theoretical requirements of the ERP properties, the corresponding multi-domain feature can be regarded as the desired feature.

Figure 4.4 shows an example of the three components in each mode to study the MMN. Figure 4.5 shows the grand averaged difference wave (DW) of the MMN in the dataset. The DW shows that the peak latency of the MMN in the dataset is approximately 150 ms. Furthermore, Figure 4.6 shows the TFR of the DW shown in Figure 4.5. The maximal power of the MMN occurs at around 5 Hz. Such temporal and spectral properties can be easily achieved. Using these properties, we can select the feature

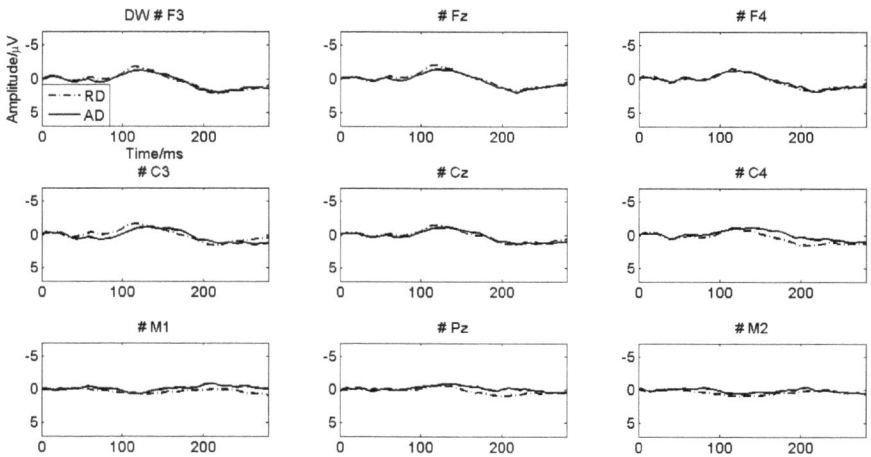

Figure 4.5   Grand averaged DW of the MMN of the children [adapted from Cong. Phan, Zhao, Huttunen-Scott, *et al.* (2012)].

#20 as the desired multi-domain feature of the MMN shown in Figure 4.4 because the corresponding temporal and spectral components meet the MMN property requirements.

4.3.3.3 *Group-level analysis of the multi-domain feature of an ERP*

After feature #20 in Figure 4.4 is selected, one-way ANOVA can be applied to determine whether the difference between the two groups is significant or not. Here, only the one-factor statistical analysis is applied because the feature mode includes only one factor "group."

If both the "group (of participants)" and "stimulus type" factors are included, the two-factor statistical analysis can be applied. Figure 4.7 shows an example (Cong *et al.*, 2014). Here, the ERP is N170, elicited by a passive oddball paradigm with the facial expressions shown in Figure 1.1. The feature mode includes two groups (control participants and participants with depression symptoms) and two stimuli (fearful and happy faces). Therefore, the two-factor statistical analysis can be applied to analyze the multi-domain feature of N170.

The ANOVA assumes that all sample populations are normally distributed, all sample populations have equal variance, and all observations are mutually independent (Hogg & Ledolter, 1987). Because of some

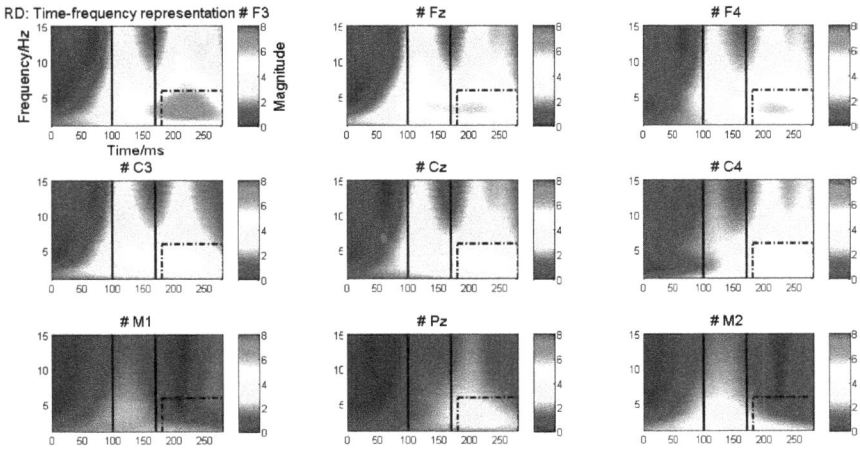

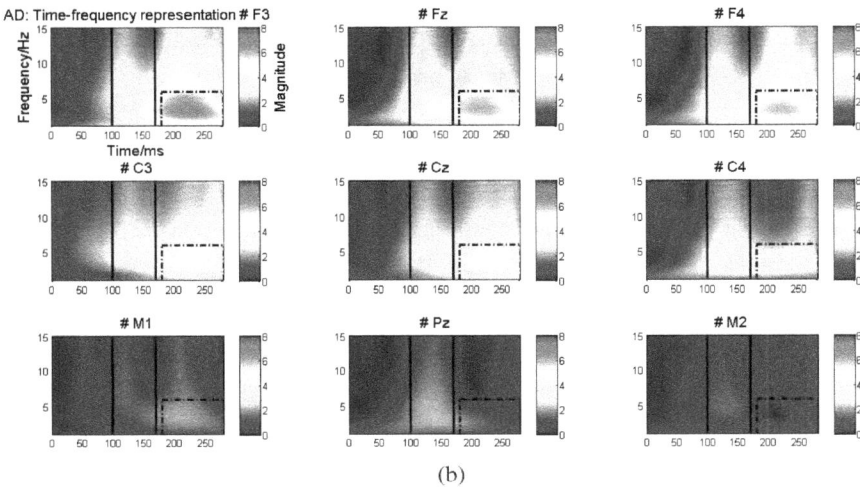

Figure 4.6   TFR of the DW shown in Figure 4.5. (a) RD. (b) AD [adapted from Cong, Phan, Zhao, Huttunen-Scott, *et al.* (2012)].

outliers, the multi-domain feature component might not meet the ANOVA assumptions. In this case, the Kruskal–Wallis test is better in determining the difference between two groups or tasks (Hogg & Ledolter, 1987; Morup *et al.*, 2007). The difference between the ANOVA and Kruskal–Wallis test is that when the data conform to the above assumptions, the

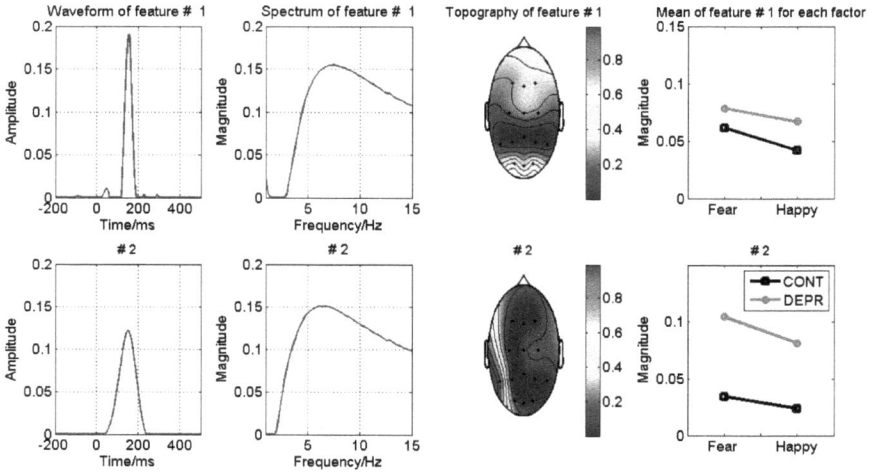

Figure 4.7   Example of NCPD on a fourth-order ERP tensor of the TFRs. The sizes of the tensor are 700 (temporal samples) × 71 (frequency bins) × 14 (channels) × 100 (composed of two groups of participants and two stimuli. The participants are 21 adults for the control and 29 adults with depression symptoms in the two groups). $R = 50$ for the NCPD, i.e., 50 components are extracted in each mode. Two of the 50 components are shown in each mode. The order of the components and the variance in a component in the NCPD are not determined. CONT: control. DEPR: depressive [adapted from Cong, *et al.* (2014)].

ANOVA test is more sensitive to the group difference; however, when the data include outliers, the nonparametric procedure, e.g., Kruskal–Wallis test, is not severely affected in determining the group difference (Hogg & Ledolter, 1987).

4.3.3.4 *Drawback in using the fourth-order ERP tensor of TFRs*

When the NCPD extracts the multi-domain feature of the ERP from the fourth-order ERP tensor that includes the time, frequency, space, and feature modes, the different subjects share the same component matrices in the time, frequency, and spatial domains. In practice, this limitation is very strong.

Furthermore, such fourth-order tensor prevents examination of the factors in the hemisphere or region along the scalp for statistical test, limiting the analysis to two factors [i.e., group of participants and stimulus type (or task)] (Cong *et al.*, 2014): the stimulus-type factor (Cong, Phan, *et al.*, 2013) and the group of participant factor (Cong, Phan, Zhao, Huttunen-Scott, *et al.*, 2012).

In actual ERP studies, the statistical analysis tends to involve two or multiple factors. In particular, the hemisphere factor in the ERPs is important. From this perspective, we need to formulate new ERP tensors of the TFRs to extract the multi-domain feature of ERPs.

4.3.4 Multi-domain feature of ERPs extracted by NCPD from a third-order ERP tensor of the TFRs

When a third-order ERP tensor of the TFRs includes the time, frequency, and feature modes (the feature mode can include the "participant," "stimulus," and "space"), it can be decomposed by the NCPD into three component matrices of the three modes as follows:

$$\underline{\mathbf{X}} = \underline{\mathbf{I}} \times_1 \mathbf{U}^{(t)} \times_2 \mathbf{U}^{(s)} \times_3 \mathbf{F} + \underline{\mathbf{E}} = \sum_{r=1}^{R} \mathbf{u}_r^{(t)} \circ \mathbf{u}_r^{(s)} \circ \mathbf{f}_r + \underline{\mathbf{E}}, \qquad (4\text{-}11)$$

where $\mathbf{U}^{(t)} = [\mathbf{u}_1^{(t)}, \mathbf{u}_2^{(t)}, \ldots, \mathbf{u}_R^{(t)}] \in \Re^{I_t \times R}$ denotes the temporal component matrix, $\mathbf{U}^{(s)} = [\mathbf{u}_1^{(s)}, \mathbf{u}_2^{(s)}, \ldots, \mathbf{u}_R^{(s)}] \in \Re^{I_s \times R}$ represents the spectral component matrix, and $\mathbf{F} = [\mathbf{f}_1, \mathbf{f}_2, \ldots, \mathbf{f}_R] \in \Re^{I \times R}$ denotes the multi-domain feature component matrix.

Figure 4.8 shows an example of the NCPD on a third-order ERP tensor of the TFRs that includes the time, frequency, and feature modes. The ERP data are obtained from the previous study of the MMN of children (Cong, Phan, Zhao, Huttunen-Scott, *et al.*, 2012). In this example, $R = 36$ in Eq. (4-11), and the ERP data of the two electrodes at two hemispheres (C3 and C4) and the two groups of children are used to formulate the third-order tensor. In the feature mode, two factors, namely, hemisphere and group, are used for the two-factor statistical analysis. In this example, the P3a components (Escera, Yago, & Alho, 2001; Huttunen-Scott, Kaartinen, Tolvanen, & Lyytinen, 2008; Huttunen, Halonen, Kaartinen, & Lyytinen, 2007), shown at the bottom row in Figure 4.8, are extracted.

Figure 4.9 shows another example of the NCPD on a third-order ERP tensor of the TFRs that includes the time, frequency, and feature modes. The ERP data are obtained from the previous study of N170 of adults. In this

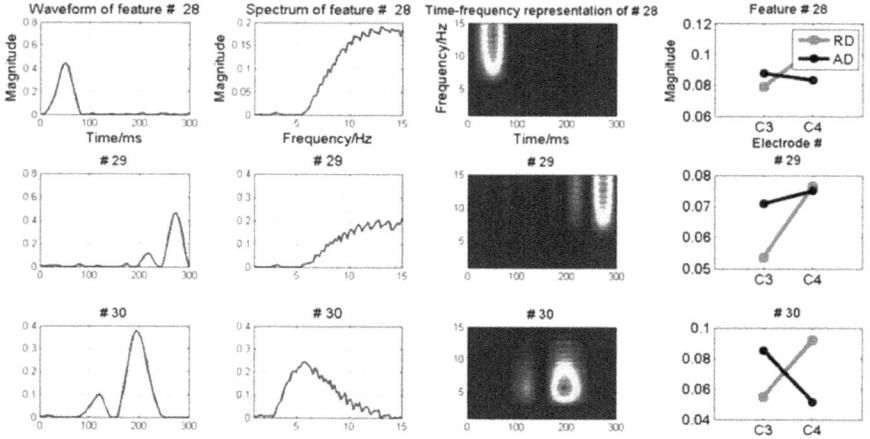

Figure 4.8   Example of NCPD on a third-order ERP tensor of the TFRs. The sizes of the tensor are 60 (temporal samples) × 71 (frequency bins) × 84 (the subjects include two groups of children and two electrode locations. Each group consists of 21 children. The two electrode locations are at C3 and C4, which are typical for MMN study). $R = 36$ for the NCPD, i.e., 36 components are extracted from each mode. Three of the 36 components are shown in each mode. The order of the components and the variance in a component in the NCPD are not determined. RD: reading disability. AD: attention deficit. The TFR in the third column is based on the outer product of the temporal and spectral components. The ERP data are from Cong, Phan, Zhao, Huttunen-Scott, *et al.* (2012).

example, $R = 31$ in Eq. (4-11). The ERP data of the two electrodes at two hemispheres (P7 and P8), two deviant and two standard stimuli, and two adult groups are used to formulate the third-order tensor. In the feature mode, the hemisphere, stimulus-type, and group factors are used for the three-factor statistical analysis.

4.3.5 *Multi-domain feature of an ERP extracted by NTD*

When a fourth-order ERP tensor of the TFRs includes the time, frequency, space, and subject modes (the subject mode can include the "participant" and "stimulus"), it can be decomposed by NTD into four component matrices of the four modes and a core tensor as follows:

$$\underline{\mathbf{X}} = \underline{\mathbf{F}} \times_1 \mathbf{A}^{(t)} \times_2 \mathbf{A}^{(s)} \times_3 \mathbf{A}^{(c)} + \underline{\mathbf{E}}, \tag{4-12}$$

where $\mathbf{A}^{(t)} = [\mathbf{a}_1^{(t)}, \mathbf{a}_2^{(t)}, \ldots, \mathbf{a}_{R_t}^{(t)}] \in \Re^{I_t \times R_t}$ denotes the temporal component matrix, $\mathbf{A}^{(s)} = [\mathbf{a}_1^{(s)}, \mathbf{a}_2^{(s)}, \ldots, \mathbf{a}_{R_s}^{(s)}] \in \Re^{I_t \times R_s}$ represents the spectral

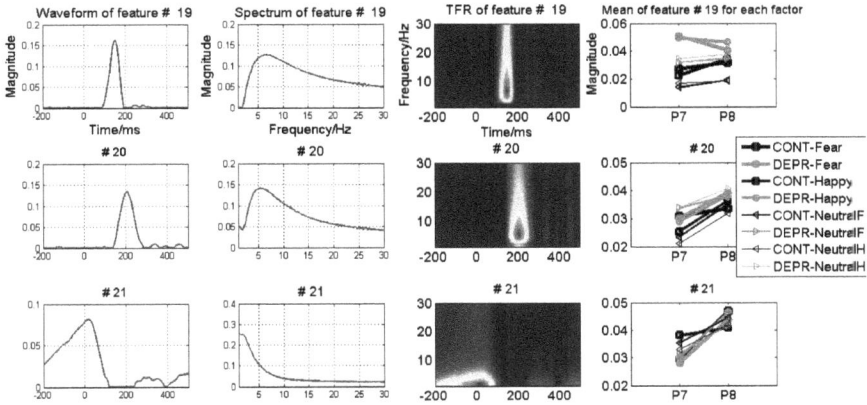

Figure 4.9 Example of NCPD on a third-order ERP tensor of the TFRs. The sizes of the tensor are 700 (temporal samples) × 141 (frequency bins) × 400 (the subjects include two adult groups, two electrode locations, and four stimulus types. The participants are composed of 21 adults for the control and 29 adults with depression symptoms in the two groups. The two electrode locations are at P7 and P8, which are typical for the N170 study). $R = 31$ for the NCPD, i.e., 31 components are extracted from each mode. Three of the 31 components are shown in each mode. The order of the components and the variance in a component in the NCPD are not determined. CONT: control. DEPR: depressive. The experimental paradigm is expressed following that shown in Figure 1.1. The TFR in the third column is based on the outer product of the temporal and spectral components. The ERP data are from Cong *et al.* (2014).

component matrix, $\mathbf{A}^{(c)} = [\mathbf{a}_1^{(c)}, \mathbf{a}_2^{(c)}, \ldots, \mathbf{a}_{R_t}^{(c)}] \in \Re^{I_t \times R_c}$ denotes the spatial component matrix, and $\underline{\mathbf{F}} \in \underline{\Re}^{R_t \times R_s \times R_c \times I}$ represents the core tensor and contains the multi-domain features of the ERPs.

Figure 4.10 shows an example of NTD on a fourth-order ERP tensor of the TFR that includes the time, frequency, space, and subject modes. Figure 4.11 shows all the extracted multi-domain features from the fourth-order ERP tensor of the TFRs on the basis of the three component matrices of the time, frequency, and space modes. The number of all features is $105(7 \times 3 \times 5)$. The ERP data are from a previous study on the MMN of children (Cong, Phan, Zhao, Huttunen-Scott, *et al.*, 2012). Similar to the NCPD on a fourth-order tensor, the temporal, spectral, and spatial component matrices do not contain any information on the individual subjects, and they are common to all features. Variability among individual subjects exists in the core tensor.

(a)

(b)   (c)

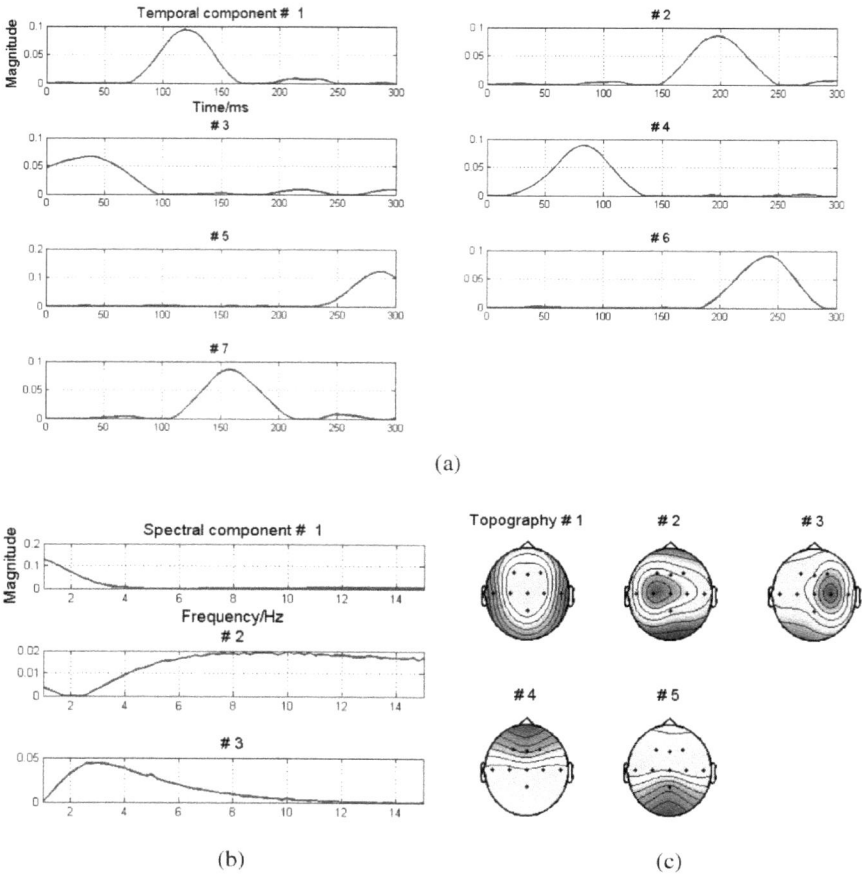

Figure 4.10   Example of NTD on a fourth-order ERP tensor of the TFRs. The sizes of the tensor are 60 (temporal samples) $\times$ 71 (frequency bins) $\times$ 9 (channels) $\times$ 42 (the subjects include two groups with 21 children per group). $R_t = 7$, $R_s = 3$, and $R_c = 5$ for the NTD, i.e., seven temporal, three spectral, and five spatial components are respectively extracted in the time, frequency, and space modes. The order of the components and the variance in a component in the NTD are not determined. The ERP data are from Cong, Phan, Zhao, Huttunen-Scott, *et al.* (2012).

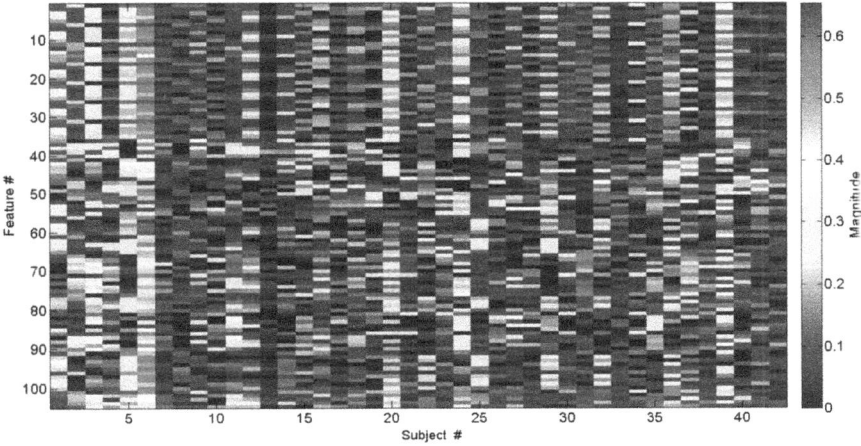

Figure 4.11 All extracted multi-domain features from the fourth-order ERP tensor of the TFRs in terms of the three component matrices of the time, frequency, and space modes.

After one component from the temporal, spectral, and spatial components is chosen, the selected multi-domain feature of the ERP is expressed as

$$\mathbf{f}_{r_t r_s r_c} = \underline{\mathbf{F}}(r_t, r_s, r_c, :). \qquad (4\text{-}13)$$

The selection of the component from each component matrix is also in accordance with a prior knowledge of the ERP of interest. For example, temporal component #7, spectral component #3, and spatial component #2 in Figure 4.10 are selected because they correspond to the MMN properties in the time, frequency, and spatial domains. They are learned from the DW, TFR, and NCPD on a fourth-order ERP tensor of the TFRs.

From Eq. (4-13), we obtain the desired multi-domain feature of the MMN shown in Figure 4.12. Then, a statistical test can be applied on the feature to examine the experimental effect. Here, only the one-factor analysis can be implemented. To analyze the multi-factor effects, NTD should be performed on the third-order ERP tensor of the TFRs, as introduced in Section 4.3.4.

We note that NTD is performed according to the Tucker model, and any component in any component matrix can interact with one another.

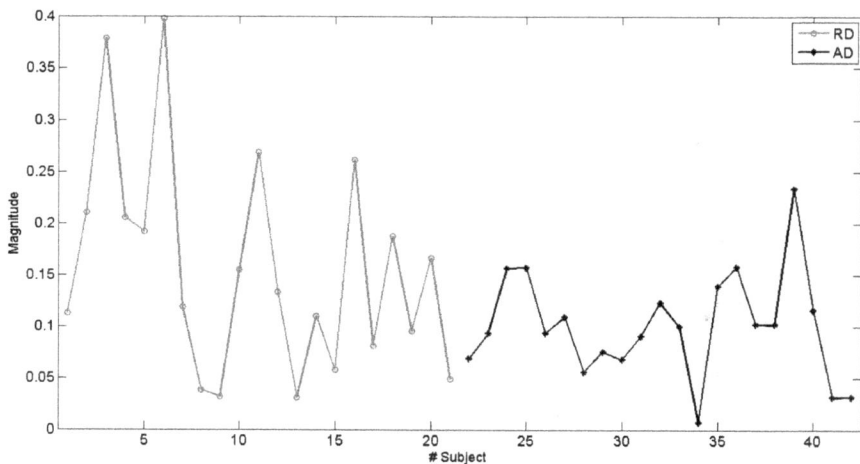

(a)

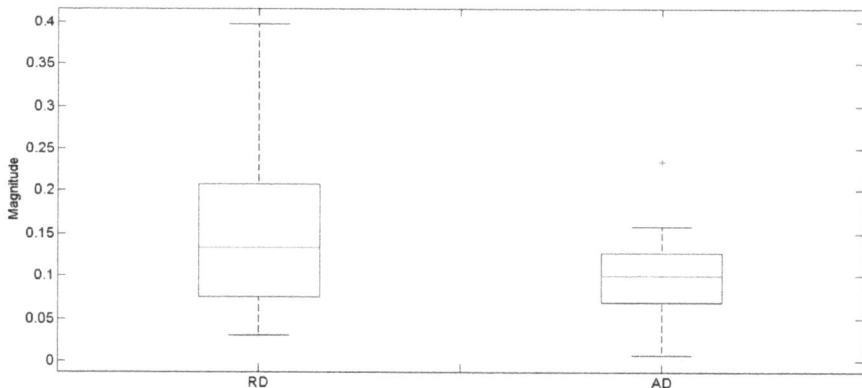

(b)

Figure 4.12   Desired multi-domain feature of the MMN extracted by NTD from the fourth-order ERP tensor of the TFRs that include the time, frequency, space, and subject modes. (a) Feature component. (b) Box plot of the feature for the two groups of children. The ERP data are obtained from Cong, Phan, Zhao, Huttunen-Scott, *et al.* (2012).

Figure 4.10 shows that any temporal component in (a), any spectral component in (b), and any spatial component in (c) can interact, which is very different from the relationship among the components of the different modes in the NCPD. In Figure 4.4, for example, only the components in the same row are associated with one another.

4.3.6 *Third-order ERP tensor of the TFRs for NTF*

4.3.6.1 *ERP tensor of the TFRs for individual topographies*

In Section 4.3.4, we introduced the third-order ERP tensor of the TFRs for NCPD that includes the time, frequency, and feature modes. In particular, the feature mode can include the group of participants, stimulus type, and hemisphere factors. In this tensor, the space and subject modes are merged, which allows testing the individual ERP spatial properties among different subjects. Other methods are also available that organize the third-order ERP tensors of TFRs. They are introduced in the next sections.

4.3.6.2 *ERP tensor of the TFRs for individual temporal components*

If the time and subject modes are merged, the third-order ERP tensor of the TFRs for NCPD includes the frequency, space, and feature modes. Therefore, investigating the individual temporal properties of the ERP among different subjects can be performed.

4.3.6.3 *ERP tensor of the TFRs for individual spectra*

Similarly, the third-order ERP tensor of the TFRs for NCPD with the time, space, and feature modes can be formulated provided that the frequency and subject modes are merged. Then, the spectral properties of the individuals remain after NCPD is applied on the ERP tensor.

In addition to the NCPD, the third-order ERP tensors of the TFRs can also be decomposed by NTD, but the features are carried by the core tensor instead of a component matrix in the NCPD.

4.3.7 *Uniqueness analysis*

In practice, we find that the variant of the Kruskal's theorem (introduced in Section 4.2.3.3) is always met with the appropriate number of components when NCPD is applied on the ERP tensor of the TFRs of the averaged EEG data (Cong *et al.*, 2014).

For the NTD on the ERP tensor of the TFRs with appropriate numbers of components in all modes, it is surprising that the uniqueness for NTD is almost met because of the applied nonnegative constraint (Zhou & Cichocki, 2012).

4.4 Adaptive and Objective Extraction of ROI from the TFRs of the ERPs

Section 4.1.1.3 introduced that the original motivation in applying the NTF on the ERP tensor of the TFRs is to objectively extract the ROIs of the TFRs. In Figures 4.8 and 4.9, the TFR (derived in terms of the outer product of the temporal and spectral components) indicates that the ROIs of the MMN and P3a are adaptively and objectively extracted. This result shows that the NTF can be a very good tool in analyzing the ERPs represented in the time-frequency domain.

Because of the variance indeterminacy of the extracted component by the NTF, determining the group-level effects of the ERP experiments will be very difficult if the NTF is applied on each ERP data of the subject. This condition is the key difference between the individual measurement of ROI using the rectangle shown in Figure 4.1 and the extraction of ROI by NTF from the grouped data.

Chapter 3 presented that the variance and polarity indeterminacies of an independent component extracted by ICA can be completely corrected under the global optimization of the ICA decomposition (Cong, Kalyakin, & Ristaniemi, 2011; Cong, Kalyakin, Zheng, & Ristaniemi, 2011). However, correcting the variance and polarity indeterminacies of a component extracted by NTF has not been theoretically made possible until now.

4.5 Key Issues in Using the NTF to Extract the Multi-Domain Feature of an ERP from the ERP Tensor of the TFRs

4.5.1 *LRA-based fast NTF algorithm*

The current trend in cognitive neuroscience research using ERPs in the EEG is to utilize a high-density sensor array and high sampling frequency in the data collection. For group-level analysis of the ERPs, the aforementioned high-order ERP tensor data can be large (e.g., hundreds of megabytes). This condition makes the benchmark tensor decomposition algorithms, e.g., the ALS (Bro, 1998), multiplicative approaches (Lee & Seung, 1999), and HALS (Cichocki *et al.*, 2007), very slow in decomposing the data.

Recently, LRA-based NTF algorithms for both the CP and Tucker models have been developed (Cong *et al.*, 2014; Zhou *et al.*, 2012). Without losing accuracy, the new algorithms are much more computationally efficient than the benchmark algorithms (Cong *et al.*, 2014; Zhou *et al.*, 2012). Indeed, NTF is based on the NMF (Cichocki *et al.*, 2009; Zhou & Cichocki, 2012). Hence, the LRA-based NMF (LRANMF) (Zhou *et al.*, 2012) is introduced as follows: for a given large-scale nonnegative matrix $\mathbf{X} \in \mathfrak{R}_+^{M \times N}$, NMF finds the basis matrix $\mathbf{A} \in \mathfrak{R}_+^{M \times R}$ and encoding matrix $\mathbf{B} \in \mathfrak{R}_+^{N \times R}$ by minimizing distance $D(\mathbf{A}, \mathbf{B}) = \|\mathbf{X} - \mathbf{AB}^T\|_F^2$.

The LRANMF conforms to the cost function expression

$$D(\tilde{\mathbf{A}}, \tilde{\mathbf{B}}; \mathbf{A}, \mathbf{B}) = \|\mathbf{X} - \tilde{\mathbf{A}}\tilde{\mathbf{B}}^T\|_F^2 + \|\tilde{\mathbf{A}}\tilde{\mathbf{B}}^T - \mathbf{AB}^T\|_F^2,$$

where $\tilde{\mathbf{A}} \in \mathfrak{R}_+^{M \times P}$, $\tilde{\mathbf{B}} \in \mathfrak{R}_+^{N \times P}$, $M \leq N$, and $P = \mu R \ll M$, and $\mu \geq 1$ is a small positive constant and typically set to one for the standard NMF.

Minimizing the above cost function usually includes two steps (Zhou *et al.*, 2012) as follows:

(1) LRA by minimizing $\|\mathbf{X} - \tilde{\mathbf{A}}\tilde{\mathbf{B}}^T\|_F^2$.
(2) NMF for $\|\tilde{\mathbf{A}}\tilde{\mathbf{B}}^T - \mathbf{AB}^T\|_F^2$ with fixed $\tilde{\mathbf{A}}$ and $\tilde{\mathbf{B}}$.

In LRANMF, the original large matrix $\mathbf{X}$ is iteratively replaced by two much smaller matrices $\tilde{\mathbf{A}}$ and $\tilde{\mathbf{B}}$, which provides significantly reduced computational complexity. Moreover, the LRA procedure can remove the noise to some extent.

With the LRA application, the size of a mode can be dramatically reduced if this mode carries redundant information. Because the EEG data are usually collected by a very high sampling frequency, redundant information certainly exists in the EEG. For group-level data analysis, multiple participants can also share similar information. Therefore, a large space is available in the EEG data for using the LRA-based NTF algorithms to improve the computational efficiency.

4.5.2 *Determining the number of extracted components*

When tensor decomposition is applied, one critical issue is the selection of the number of components to be extracted in each mode. As expressed in Eq. (4-2), one parameter should be chosen for the CPD. However, for the Tucker decomposition, the selection becomes more complicated and usually, the numbers of components for the different modes in Eq. (4-5) are different.

4.5.2.1 *MOS*

Actually, choosing the number of components to be extracted is an inherent problem in model order selection (MOS). This is usually applied in the over-determined linear transform model, i.e., the number of sensors that collect the data is greater than the number of sources, as introduced in Section 3.5. Indeed, the methods described in that subsection are for matrix decomposition. Therefore, we need to reshape the tensor into a matrix to apply these methods. Subsequently, the number of components can be estimated by the MOS methods (He, Cichocki, & Xie, 2009; He, Cichocki, Xie, & Choi, 2010). This approach depends on how the tensor is very well reshaped for the real-world physical data (He *et al.*, 2010) and signal-to-noise ratio (SNR) level of the data (Cong, Nandi, He, Cichocki, & Ristaniemi, 2012).

Sometimes, selection of the number of components is based on the percentage of the explained variance using a certain number of eigenvalues over all eigenvalues instead of the MOS methods in terms of the specially designed eigenspectrum illustrated in Section 3.5. The eigenvalues belong to the sample covariance of the matrix, which is derived from the reshaped tensor.

4.5.2.2 *ARD*

Recently, a Bayesian learning-based method, which is called automatic relevance determination (ARD), has been proposed to determine the number of components in each mode in tensor decomposition (Morup & Hansen, 2009). ARD belongs to the hierarchical Bayesian approach and has been used for model selection (Morup & Hansen, 2009). In ARD, the relevance of the different extracted components can be explicitly represented by hyperparameters, the range of variation of these components may be defined, and the width of the zero-mean Gaussian imposed on the model parameters can be modeled (Morup & Hansen, 2009). In case the width is zero, no effect on the prediction will be induced by the corresponding component. Therefore, the hyperparameters are optimized to extract the relevant components (Morup & Hansen, 2009). The ARD software can be downloaded from the following link: www.erpwavelab.org. In this software, the number of components in each factor should be initialized.

In this book, because nonnegative constraint is added for optimization of the tensor decomposition, the prior is given by the exponential distribution (Morup & Hansen, 2009). We have learned that when the SNR is low, the ARD cannot accurately estimate the number of components to be extracted (Cong, Phan, *et al.*, 2013).

4.5.2.3 *Data-driven methods*

The data-driven methods, which include the DIFFIT (Timmerman & Kiers, 2000), CORCONDIA (Bro, Kjeldahl, Smilde, & Kiers, 2008), and cross validation (Bro *et al.*, 2008), appear to be very useful although they are very time consuming. In using these methods, a library of the numbers of components is first selected, and tensor decomposition is performed over these numbers. Subsequently, the DIFFIT and CORCONDIA respectively measure the change in the fit (explained variance of the raw data by the proposed model) and the core tensor of the decomposition among the number of models. The cross-validation method measures the change in the component matrix in each mode using different numbers of components.

We introduce DIFFIT next. The difference fit of two adjacent fits is given by

$$\text{dif}(R) = \text{fit}(R) - \text{fit}(R - 1),$$

where $R = 2, \ldots, L$. Then, the ratio of the adjacent difference fits is expressed as

$$\text{diffit}(R) = \frac{\text{dif}(R)}{\text{dif}(R + 1)},$$

where $R = 2, \ldots, L - 1$. The model with the largest diffit value is regarded as the appropriate number of components for tensor decomposition (Timmerman & Kiers, 2000).

Figure 4.13 shows an example of the DIFFIT. The fit of each selected NTD model is for a fourth-order ERP tensor of the TFRs (Cong, Phan,

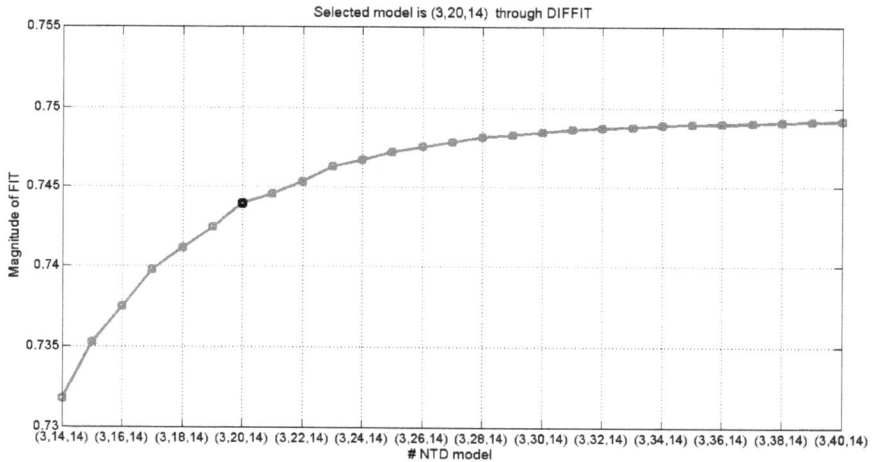

Figure 4.13   Fits of the different NTD models [adapted from Cong *et al.* (2013)].

et al., 2013). It changes over the number of temporal components. In this example, the numbers of spectral and spatial components are fixed to 3 and 14, respectively, aimed at determining the appropriate number of temporal components. After the DIFFIT is applied, "20" is proposed because the increase in the fit is maximal for this NTD model. Thus, DIFFIT is applied to measure the saturation of the fit.

4.5.3 *Stability of the multi-domain feature of the ERP extracted by the NTF*

Similar to ICA algorithms, most NTF algorithms are also adaptive. Therefore, we need to evaluate if the decomposed results are stable or not. The commonly used method is to examine the change in the fits when NTF is run multiple times on the same model (Cichocki *et al.*, 2009).

Sections 4.2.3 and 4.2.4 presented that both the CPD and Tucker decomposition are the sum of a number of rank-one tensors plus the additive noise tensor. Motivated by this tensor decomposition characteristic, we proposed an effective method in our previous studies (Cong, Phan, *et al.*, 2013; Cong, Phan, Zhao, Huttunen-Scott, *et al.*, 2012; Cong *et al.*, 2014). The new method is expressed in terms of the correlation coefficient between the template rank-one tensor and each extracted rank-one tensor to investigate the stability of the extracted multi-domain feature of the ERP by the NTF.

We consider an example of NCPD on a fourth-order ERP tensor of the TFRs that includes the time, frequency, space, and feature modes. After the appropriate number of components is determined by DIFFIT, the desired temporal, spectral, spatial, and feature components can be selected. Subsequently, a rank-one fourth-order tensor can be formulated as a template rank-one tensor.

$$\underline{\mathbf{X}}_{\text{template}} = \mathbf{u}_{\text{template}}^{(t)} \circ \mathbf{u}_{\text{template}}^{(s)} \circ \mathbf{u}_{\text{template}}^{(c)} \circ \mathbf{f}_{\text{template}}. \tag{4-14}$$

Using $\underline{\mathbf{X}}_{\text{template}}$, we examine whether the template rank-one tensor can be extracted by other NCPD models or whether it can be stably extracted when one NCPD model is run multiple times with random initialization for the component matrices.

From Eq. (4-2), each rank-one tensor in the NCPD model in each round of decomposition is correlated with the template rank-one tensor.

$$\rho(r, R, k) = [(\mathbf{u}_{(r,R,k)}^{(t)})^T \mathbf{u}_{\text{template}}^{(t)}] \cdot [(\mathbf{u}_{(r,R,k)}^{(s)})^T \mathbf{u}_{\text{template}}^{(s)}]$$
$$\cdot [(\mathbf{u}_{(r,R,k)}^{(c)})^T \mathbf{u}_{\text{template}}^{(c)}] \cdot [(\mathbf{f}_{(r,R,k)})^T \mathbf{f}_{\text{template}}], \tag{4-15}$$

where $R = 2, 3, \ldots, L$, $r = 1, \ldots, R$, and $k = 1, 2, \ldots, K$. R is the number of extracted components from each mode by the NCPD, L is the upper bound of the library of numbers of components, and K is the number of rounds to perform NCPD with random initialization in each round. Each component is normalized to its standard deviation, and its nonzero mean is subtracted before the correlation analysis. When R components are extracted in the kth round, R correlation coefficients are obtained using Eq. (4-15). Then, the maximal coefficient among the R coefficients is chosen as

$$q(R, k) = \max[\rho(1, R, k), \rho(2, R, k), \ldots, \rho(R, R, k)]. \tag{4-16}$$

Figure 4.14 shows $q(R, k)$ when NCPD is applied on a fourth-order EPR tensor of the TFRs that includes the time, frequency, space, and feature modes (Cong *et al.*, 2014). This figure shows that the desired multi-domain feature of the ERP is hard to extract when the number of components R

is smaller than 15. The desired multi-domain feature of the ERP can be extracted when R ranges from approximately 50 to 60.

4.5.4 *How many components can be appropriately extracted by the NTF with knowledge of ERPs taken into account?*

When NTF is used to decompose the ERP tensor of the TFRs, BSS is achieved (Cichocki *et al.*, 2009), which is similar to the ICA on the EEG data. The difference is that NTF is performed on the TFRs of the waveforms, whereas ICA is performed on the waveforms. Following this context, the number of sources in the time domain can be considered a reasonable reference in choosing the number of components to be extracted by the NTF.

In the time domain, after the preprocessing of the ERPs and applying the wavelet filter on the averaged EEG, the number of sources can be dramatically reduced to a few dozens (Cong, He, Hämäläinen, Cichocki, & Ristaniemi, 2011; Cong, He, *et al.*, 2013). The wavelet filter and TFR are two methods as the representations of the wavelet transform. Therefore, the number of sources in the TFR of the ERPs can also be reduced, in contrast to that in the ordinarily averaged EEG data. This means that the NTF cannot achieve satisfactory separation of the EEG data in the time-frequency domain when only a few components are used. For example, when ICA is applied to decompose the EEG data, a small number of components are seldom chosen. Before our studies (Cong, Phan, *et al.*, 2013; Cong, Phan, Zhao, Huttunen-Scott, *et al.*, 2012; Cong *et al.*, 2014), this fact has not been recognized when NTF or CPD was applied on high-order tensors of the EEG data. In the example shown in Figure 4.14, obtaining reasonable components is very difficult when the number of components is few.

We recommend that the estimated number of sources in the averaged EEG data should be taken into account when selecting the number of temporal components to be extracted by the NCPD and NTD from the ERP tensor of the TFRs. This number is usually a few dozens. From our empirical knowledge, the number of spectral and spatial components to be extracted by the NTD can be much smaller than the number of temporal components (Cong, Phan, *et al.*, 2013) because the ERP data dynamics in the frequency and spatial domains are fewer than that in the time domain.

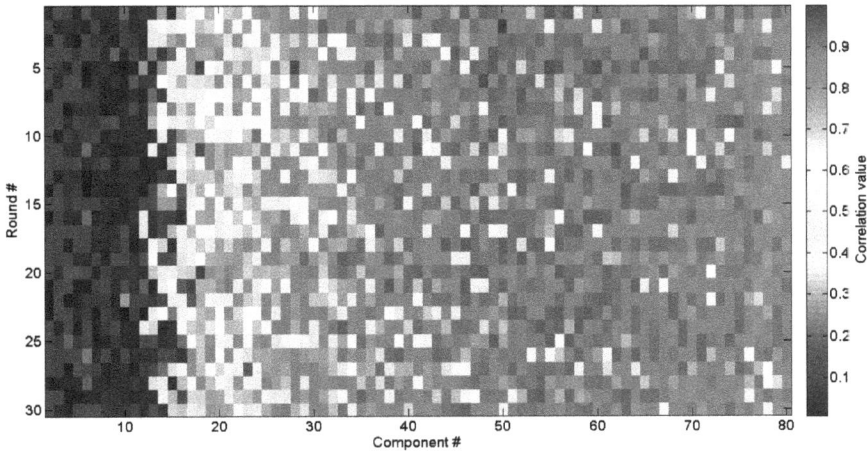

Figure 4.14 Stability analysis of the results of the NCPD on the ERP tensor of the TFRs. The tensor is used for the results shown in Figure 4.7. The four components in the second row in Figure 4.7 compose the template rank-one tensor of Eq. (4-15), which produces the results here [adapted from Cong *et al.* (2014)].

4.5.5 *Which tensor decomposition model should be chosen for the NTF?*

The CP and Tucker models are two major models for tensor decomposition. In order for the NTF to extract the multi-domain feature of the ERP, the NCPD is more straightforward for feature selection than the NTD, and determining the number of extracted components is much simpler. These models were presented in Sections 4.3.3–4.3.5. Nevertheless, the advantage of the NTD is that the Tucker model offers more possibilities in decomposing a tensor. In addition to these theoretical analyses, we need to consider the SNR of the data in practice.

When the SNR of the averaged EEG data is high enough, we recommend using the NCPD to extract the multi-domain feature of the ERP from the ERP tensor of the TFRs. As an example, the same fourth-order ERP tensor of the TFRs is decomposed by the NCPD and NTD, and the results of both methods are shown in Figures 4.4 and 4.10, respectively. Both the NCPD and NTD produce satisfactory results. However, when the SNR of the averaged EEG data is low, we recommend using the NTD, instead of the NCPD, to extract the multi-domain feature of the ERP from the ERP tensor of the

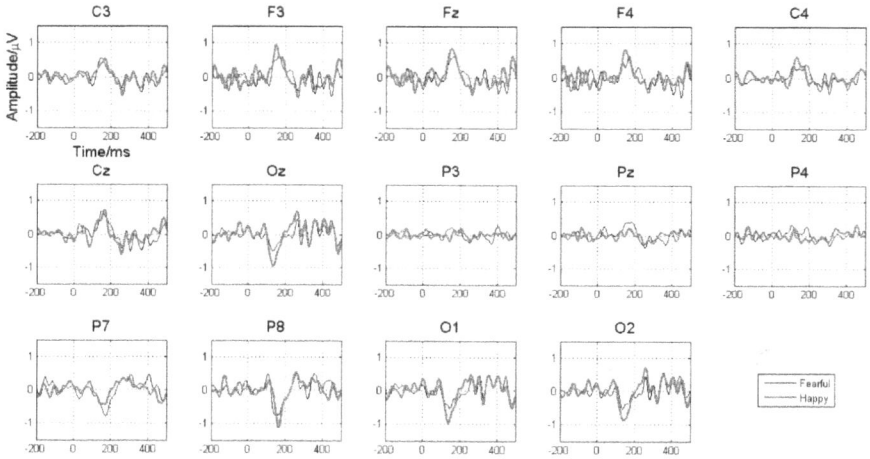

Figure 4.15 Grand averaged DW waveforms. The experimental paradigm is shown in Figure 1.1 [adapted from Cong, Phan, *et al.* (2013)].

TFRs. This is because the Tucker model is more powerful in decomposing the mixture into individual components. Figure 4.15 shows a noisy ERP, which is a visual MMN (vMMN) (Cong, Phan, *et al.*, 2013). The grand averaged EEG data in the figure are grand averaged DWs. The ERP data are clearly very noisy. Figure 4.16 shows the results of the NCPD on a fourth-order vMMN tensor of the TFRs that includes the time, frequency, space, and feature modes (Cong, Phan, *et al.*, 2013). From the BSS viewpoint, the mixture is not well separated into individual components compared with those shown in Figures 4.4 and 4.7–4.9.

Figure 4.17 shows the temporal, spectral, and spatial components extracted by the NTD in terms of Eq. (4-12) (Cong, Phan, *et al.*, 2013). Even though the vMMN data are very noisy, the NTD still satisfactorily extracts the components in each mode from the BSS viewpoint. Moreover, the multi-domain vMMN feature extracted by the NTD satisfies more the theoretical expectations than that by the NCPD in terms of the psychophysiological vMMN knowledge (Cong, Phan, *et al.*, 2013).

4.6 Summary

In the application of the NTF on the fourth- or third-order ERP tensor of the TFRs, the tensor is simultaneously filtered by the NTF in the time, frequency,

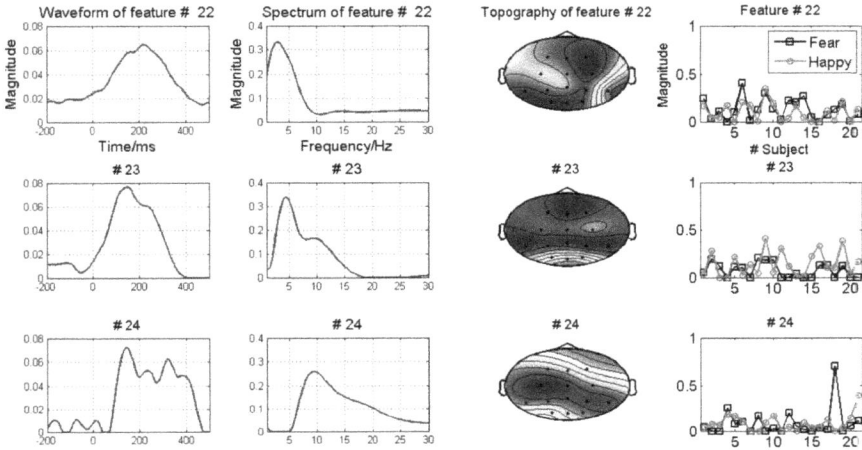

Figure 4.16 Example of the NCPD on a fourth-order vMMN tensor of the TFRs. The sizes of the tensor are 700 (temporal samples) × 59 (frequency bins) × 14 (channels) × 42 (21 adults and two stimuli). $R = 32$ for the NCPD, i.e., 32 components are extracted from each mode. Three of the 32 components are shown in each mode. The order of the components and the variance in a component in the NCPD are not determined [adapted from Cong, Phan, *et al.* (2013)].

space, and subject domains. The multi-domain feature of the ERP extracted by the NTF from the ERP tensor of the TFRs is a new biomarker for cognitive neuroscience research. It reveals the strength of the brain activity elicited by the stimuli. This new feature is particularly suitable for group-level analysis of the ERPs and can be used in multiple-factor statistical analysis such as the ERP peak amplitude. Figures 4.4 and 4.7– 4.10 show that the feature-carrying variability of the different subjects is determined in terms of the common subspaces across the different subjects in all or some parts of the time, frequency, and space domains. The common subspaces depend on how the ERP tensor of the TFRs for the NTF is organized, which was discussed in Section 4.3.6.

In summary, the new approach for group-level analysis of the ERPs using the multi-domain feature of the ERP includes the following seven steps:

(1) Preprocessing of the single-trial EEG data and averaging the preprocessed EEG data over single trials.
(2) Performing wavelet transform on the averaged EEG data to obtain the TFRs of the ERPs.

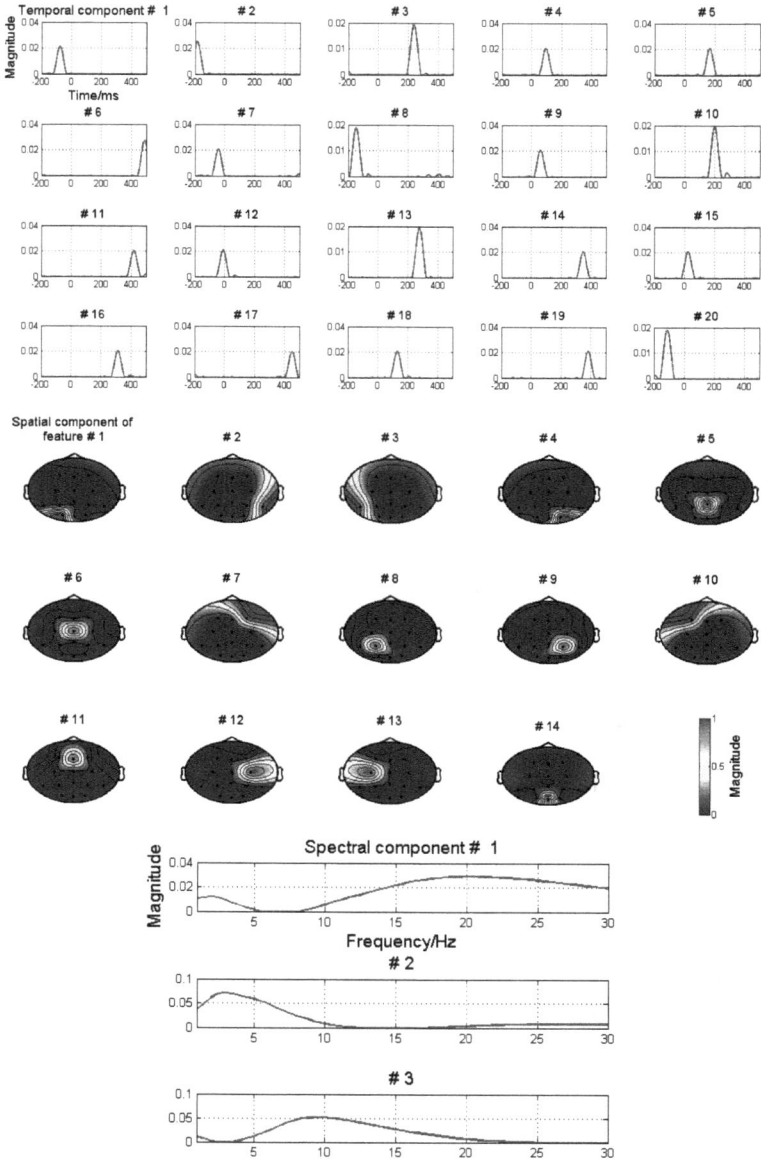

Figure 4.17   Temporal, spectral, and spatial components extracted by the NTD from the vMMN tensor of the TFRs shown in Figure 4.16 [adapted from Cong, Phan, *et al.* (2013)].

(3) Organizing the ERP tensor of the TFRs according to the research interest.

(4) Determining the number of components for each model to be extracted by the NTF.

(5) Performing the NTF to extract the multi-domain features of the ERPs from the ERP tensor of the TFRs.

(6) Selecting the desired multi-domain feature of the ERP in terms of the ERP properties in the time, frequency, and/or spatial domains (depending on how the ERP tensor is organized).

(7) Analyzing the multi-domain feature of the ERP using multi-factor statistical analysis.

4.7 Existing Key Problem and Potential Solution

In the tensor decomposition application to analyze the ERPs, how to evaluate the stability of the extracted components in different modes has not been paid enough attention until today. Indeed, this is a very critical problem. The clustering approach used in the ICA could be one solution.

4.8 MATLAB Codes

The application of tensor decomposition has been more and more popular now in the field of signal processing (Cichocki *et al.*, 2014). There are many existing MATLAB toolboxes. We list the mostly acknowledged ones as the following:

http://www.bsp.brain.riken.jp/~zhougx/tensor.html.

http://www.esat.kuleuven.be/sista/tensorlab/.

http://www.sandia.gov/~tgkolda/TensorToolbox/index-2.5.html.

http://www.models.life.ku.dk/nwaytoolbox.

www.erpwavelab.org.

Particularly, demo data in Figure 4.4 can be downloaded via http://www.escience.cn/people/cong/index.html.

In order to use those toolboxes and the demo data, one has to know how to program with MATLAB.

References

Acar, E., Aykut-Bingol, C., Bingol, H., Bro, R., & Yener, B. (2007). Multiway analysis of epilepsy tensors. *Bioinformatics (Oxford, England)*, *23*(13), i10–i18. doi: 10.1093/bioinformatics/btm210.

Acar, E., Bingol, C. A., & Bingol, H. (2006). Computational analysis of epileptic focus localization. *Proceedings of the Fourth IASTED International Conference on Biomedical Engineering*, 317–322.

Acar, E., Bingol, C. A., Bingol, H., Bro, R., & Yener, B. (2007). Seizure recognition on epilepsy feature tensor. *Conference Proceedings: Annual International Conference of the IEEE Engineering in Medicine and Biology Society. IEEE Engineering in Medicine and Biology Society. Conference*, *2007*, 4273–4276. doi: 10.1109/IEMBS.2007.4353280.

Acar, E. & Yener, B. (2009). Unsupervised multiway data analysis: A literature survey. *IEEE Transactions on Knowledge and Data Engineering*, *21*(1), 6–20.

Achim, A. & Bouchard, S. (1997). Toward a dynamic topographic components model. *Electroencephalography and Clinical Neurophysiology*, *103*, 381–385.

Adeli, H. & Ghosh-Dastidar, S. (2010). *Automated EEG-Based Diagnosis of Neurological Disorders — Inventing the Future of Neurology*. Florida, USA: CRC Press.

Axmacher, N., Cohen, M. X., Fell, J., Haupt, S., Dumpelmann, M., Elger, C. E., ... Ranganath, C. (2010). Intracranial EEG correlates of expectancy and memory formation in the human hippocampus and nucleus accumbens. *Neuron*, *65*(4), 541–549. doi: 10.1016/j.neuron.2010.02.006.

Basar, E. (2004). *Memory and Brain Dynamics: Oscillations Integrating Attention, Perception, Learning, and Memory* (Vol. 1). Florida, USA: CRC Press.

Basar, E., Schurmann, M., Demiralp, T., Basar-Eroglu, C., & Ademoglu, A. (2001). Event-related oscillations are 'real brain responses' — Wavelet analysis and new strategies. *International Journal of Psychophysiology: Official Journal of the International Organization of Psychophysiology*, *39*(2–3), 91–127.

Beckmann, C. F. & Smith, S. M. (2005). Tensorial extensions of independent component analysis for multisubject FMRI analysis. *NeuroImage*, *25*(1), 294–311. doi: 10.1016/j.neuroimage.2004.10.043.

Bertrand, O. & Tallon-Baudry, C. (2000). Oscillatory gamma activity in humans: A possible role for object representation. *International Journal of Psychophysiology: Official Journal of the International Organization of Psychophysiology*, *38*(3), 211–223.

Bishop, C. M. (2006). *Pattern Recognition and Machine Learning* (Vol. 1). Singapore: Springer.

Bishop, D. V. M. & Hardiman, M. J. (2010). Measurement of mismatch negativity in individuals: A study using single-trial analysis. *Psychophysiology*, *37*, 697–705.

Bro, R. (1998). *Multi-Way Analysis in the Food Industry — Models, Algorithms, and Applications*. PhD thesis. Holland: University of Amsterdam.

Bro, R., Kjeldahl, K., Smilde, A. K., & Kiers, H. A. L. (2008). Cross-validation of component models: A critical look at current methods. *Analytical and Bioanalytical Chemistry*, *390*, 1241–1251.

Carroll, J. D. & Chang, J. (1970). Analysis of individual differences in multidimensional scaling via an n-way generalization of 'Eckart-Young' decomposition. *Psychometrika*, *35*, 283–319.

Cavanagh, J. F., Cohen, M. X., & Allen, J. J. (2009). Prelude to and resolution of an error: EEG phase synchrony reveals cognitive control dynamics during action monitoring. *The Journal of Neuroscience: The Official Journal of the Society for Neuroscience*, *29*(1), 98–105. doi: 10.1523/JNEUROSCI.4137-08.2009.

Cichocki, A. (2013). Tensors decompositions: New concepts for brain data analysis? *Journal of Control Measurement, and System Integration*, *6*(7), 507–517.

Cichocki, A. & Amari, S. (2003). *Adaptive Blind Signal and Image Processing: Learning Algorithms and Applications* (Vol. Revised). Chichester: John Wiley & Sons Inc.

Cichocki, A., Mandic, D., Caiafa, C., Phan, A-H., Zhou, G., Zhao, Q., & De Lathauwer, L. (2014). Tensor decompositions for signal processing applications from two-way to multiway component analysis. *IEEE Signal Processing Magazine, In Press*.

Cichocki, A., Washizawa, Y., Rutkowski, T. M., Bakardjian, H., Phan, A. H., Choi, S., & Zhao, Q. (2008). Noninvasive BCIs: Multiway signal-processing array decompositions. *Computer*, *41*(10), 34–42.

Cichocki, A., Zdunek, R., & Amari, S. (2007). Hierarchical ALS Algorithms for Nonnegative Matrix and 3d Tensor Factorization. In M. E. Davies *et al.* (Eds.). ICA 2007, *Lecture Notes in Computer Science*, 4666, 169–176.

Cichocki, A., Zdunek, R., Phan, A. H., & Amari, S. (2009). *Nonnegative Matrix and Tensor Factorizations: Applications to Exploratory Multi-way Data Analysis*. John Wiley.

Cohen, M. X. (2014). *Analyzing Neural Time Series Data: Theory and Practice* Cambridge, MA: The MIT Press.

Comon, P. (1994). Independent component analysis, a new concept? *Signal Processing*, *36*(3), 287–314.

Comon, P. & Jutten, C. (2010). *Handbook of Blind Source Separation: Independent Component Analysis and Applications* (Vol. 1). Academic Press.

Cong, F., He, Z., Hämäläinen, J., Cichocki, A., & Ristaniemi, T. (2011). Determining the number of sources in high-density EEG recordings of event-related potentials by model order selection. *Proceedings of IEEE Workshop on Machine Learning for Signal Processing (MLSP) 2011*, Beijing, China, September 18–21, 1–6.

Cong, F., He, Z., Hämäläinen, J., Leppänen, P. H. T., Lyytinen, H., Cichocki, A., & Ristaniemi, T. (2013). Validating rationale of group-level component analysis based on estimating number of sources in EEG through model order selection. *Journal of Neuroscience Methods*, *212*(1), 165–172.

Cong, F., Kalyakin, I., & Ristaniemi, T. (2011). Can back-projection fully resolve polarity indeterminacy of ICA in study of ERP? *Biomedical Signal Processing and Control*, *6*(4), 422–426.

Cong, F., Kalyakin, I., Zheng, C., & Ristaniemi, T. (2011). Analysis on subtracting projection of extracted independent components from EEG recordings. *Biomedizinische Technik/Biomedical Engineering*, *56*(4), 223–234.

Cong, F., Nandi, A. K., He, Z., Cichocki, A., & Ristaniemi, T. (2012). Fast and effective model order selection method to determine the number of sources in a linear transformation model. *Proceedings of the 2012 European Signal Processing Conference (EUSIPCO-2012)*, 1870–1874.

Cong, F., Phan, A. H., Astikainen, P., Zhao, Q., Hietanen, J. K., Ristaniemi, T., & Cichocki, A. (2012). Multi-domain feature of event-related potential extracted by nonnegative tensor factorization: 5 vs. 14 electrodes EEG data. In A. Cichocki *et al.* (Eds.). LVA/ICA 2012, *Lecture Notes in Computer Science*, 7191, 502–510.

Cong, F., Phan, A. H., Astikainen, P., Zhao, Q., Wu, Q., Hietanen, J. K., ... Cichocki, A. (2013). Multi-domain feature extraction for small event-related potentials through nonnegative multi-way array decomposition from low dense array EEG. *International Journal of Neural Systems, 23* (2(1350006)), 1–18. doi: 10.1142/S012906571 3500068.

Cong, F., Phan, A. H., Zhao, Q., Huttunen-Scott, T., Kaartinen, J., Ristaniemi, T., ... Cichocki, A. (2012). Benefits of multi-domain feature of mismatch negativity extracted by non-negative tensor factorization from EEG collected by low-density array. *International Journal of Neural Systems, 22*(6–1250025), 1–19. doi: 10.1142/S0129065712500256.

Cong, F., Phan, A. H., Zhao, Q., Nandi, A. K., Alluri, V., Toiviainen, P., ... Ristaniemi, T. (2012). Analysis of ongoing EEG elicited by natural music stimuli using nonnegative tensor factorization. *Proceeding of the 2012 European Signal Processing Conference (EUSIPCO-2012)*, Bucharest, Romania, August 27–31, Bucharest, Romania, 494–498.

Cong, F., Zhou, G., Astikainen, P., Zhao, Q., Wu, Q., Nandi, A.K., ... Cichocki, A. (2014). Low-rank approximation based nonnegative multi-way array decomposition on event-related potentials. *International Journal of Neural Systems*, doi:10.1142/S012906571440005X.

Daubechies, I. (1992). *Ten Lectures on Wavelets*. Society for Industrial and Applied Mathematics.

Daubechies, I., Roussos, E., Takerkart, S., Benharrosh, M., Golden, C., D'Ardenne, K., ... Haxby, J. (2009). Independent component analysis for brain fMRI does not select for independence. *PNAS, 106*(26), 10415–10422.

David, O., Kilner, J. M., & Friston, K. J. (2006). Mechanisms of evoked and induced responses in MEG/EEG. *NeuroImage, 31*(4), 1580–1591. doi: 10.1016/ j.neuroimage.2006.02.034.

De Vos, M., De Lathauwer, L., Vanrumste, B., Van Huffel, S., & Van Paesschen, W. (2007). Canonical decomposition of ictal scalp EEG and accurate source localisation: Principles and simulation study. *Computational intelligence and neuroscience*, 58253. doi: 10.1155/2007/58253.

De Vos, M., Vergult, A., De Lathauwer, L., De Clercq, W., Van Huffel, S., Dupont, P., ... Van Paesschen, W. (2007). Canonical decomposition of ictal scalp EEG reliably detects the seizure onset zone. *NeuroImage, 37*(3), 844–854. doi: 10.1016/j.neuroimage.2007.04.041.

Debener, S., Ullsperger, M., Siegel, M., & Engel, A. K. (2006). Single-trial EEG-fMRI reveals the dynamics of cognitive function. *Trends in Cognitive Sciences, 10*(12), 558–563. doi: 10.1016/j.tics.2006.09.010.

Debener, S., Ullsperger, M., Siegel, M., Fiehler, K., von Cramon, D. Y., & Engel, A. K. (2005). Trial-by-trial coupling of concurrent electroencephalogram and functional magnetic resonance imaging identifies the dynamics of performance monitoring. *The Journal of Neuroscience: The Official Journal of the Society for Neuroscience, 25*(50), 11730–11737. doi: 10.1523/JNEUROSCI.3286-05.2005.

Deburchgraeve, W., Cherian, P., De Vos, M., Swarte, R., Blok, J., Visser, G., ... Van Huffel, S. (2009). Neonatal seizure localization using PARAFAC decomposition. *Clinical Neurophysiology: Official Journal of the International Federation of Clinical Neurophysiology, 120*, 1787–1796.

Delorme, A. & Makeig, S. (2004). EEGLAB: An open source toolbox for analysis of single-trial EEG dynamics including independent component analysis. *Journal of Neuroscience Methods, 134*(1), 9–21. doi: 10.1016/j.jneumeth.2003.10.009.

Eichele, T., Rachakonda, S., Brakedal, B., Eikeland, R., & Calhoun, V. D. (2011). EEGIFT: Group independent component analysis for event-related EEG data. *Computational Intelligence and Neuroscience, 2011*, 129365. doi: 10.1155/2011/129365.

Eliseyev, A. & Aksenova, T. (2013). Recursive N-way partial least squares for brain–computer interface. *PLoS ONE, 8*(7), e69962. doi: 10.1371/journal.pone.0069962.

Eliseyev, A., Moro, C., J., Faber., Wyss, A., Torres, N., Mestais, C., ... Aksenova, T. (2012). L1-penalized N-way PLS for subset of electrodes selection in BCI experiments. *Journal of Neural Engineering, 9*(4), 045010.

Escera, C., Yago, E., & Alho, K. (2001). Electrical responses reveal the temporal dynamics of brain events during involuntary attention switching. *The European Journal of Neuroscience, 14*(5), 877–883.

Field, A. & Graupe, D. (1991). Topographic component (parallel factor) analysis of multi-channel evoked potentials: Practical issues in trilinear spatiotemporal decomposition. *Brain Topography, 3*, 407–423.

Fuentemilla, L., Marco-Pallares, J., Munte, T. F., & Grau, C. (2008). Theta EEG oscillatory activity and auditory change detection. *Brain Research, 1220*, 93–101. doi: 10.1016/j.brainres.2007.07.079.

Gorsev, G. Y. & Basar, E. (2010). Sensory evoked and event related oscillations in Alzheimer's disease: A short review. *Cognitive Neurodynamics, 4*(4), 263–274.

Harshman, R. A. (1970). Foundations of the PARAFAC procedure: Models and conditions for an "explanatory" multi-modal factor analysis. *UCLA Working Papers in Phonetics, 16*, 1–84.

He, Z., Cichocki, A., & Xie, S. (2009). Efficient method for Tucker3 model selection. *Electronics Letters, 45*, 805–806.

He, Z., Cichocki, A., Xie, S., & Choi, K. (2010). Detecting the number of clusters in n-way probabilistic clustering. *IEEE Transactions on Pattern Analysis and Machine Intelligence, 32*(11), 2006–2021. doi: 10.1109/TPAMI.2010.15.

Herrmann, C. S., Rach, S., Vosskuhl, J., & Struber, D. (2013). Time-frequency analysis of event-related potentials: A brief tutorial. *Brain Topography*, 1–13. doi: 10.1007/s10548-013-0327-5.

Hitchcock, F. L. (1927). The expression of a tensor or a polyadic as a sum of products. *Journal of Mathematics and Physics, 6*(1), 164–189.

Hogg, R. V. & Ledolter, J. (1987). *Engineering Statistics*. New York: MacMillan.

Huttunen-Scott, T., Kaartinen, J., Tolvanen, A., & Lyytinen, H. (2008). Mismatch negativity (MMN) elicited by duration deviations in children with reading disorder, attention deficit or both. *International Journal of Psychophysiology: Official Journal of the International Organization of Psychophysiology*, *69*(1), 69–77. doi: 10.1016/j.ijpsycho.2008.03.002.

Huttunen, T., Halonen, A., Kaartinen, J., & Lyytinen, H. (2007). Does mismatch negativity show differences in reading-disabled children compared to normal children and children with attention deficit? *Developmental Neuropsychology*, *31*(3), 453–470. doi: 10.1080/87565640701229656.

Hyvarinen, A., Karhunen, J., & Oja, E. (2001). *Independent Component Analysis*. New York: John Wiley & Sons Inc.

Kolda, T. & Bader, B. (2009). Tensor decompositions and applications. *SIAM Review*, *51*(3), 455–500.

Kovacevic, N. & McIntosh, A. R. (2007). Groupwise independent component decomposition of EEG data and partial least square analysis. *NeuroImage*, *35*(3), 1103–1112. doi: 10.1016/j.neuroimage.2007.01.016.

Kroonenberg, P. M. (2008). *Applied Multiway Data Analysis*. Wiley.

Kruskal, J. B. (1977). Three-way arrays: Rank and uniqueness of trilinear decompositions, with application to arithmetic complexity and statistics. *Linear Algebra and its Applications*, *18*, 95–138.

Lee, D. D. & Seung, H. S. (1999). Learning the parts of objects by non-negative matrix factorization. *Nature*, *401*(6755), 788–791. doi: 10.1038/44565.

Luck, S. J. (2005). *An Introduction to the Event-Related Potential Technique*. Cambridge, MA: The MIT Press.

Miwakeichi, F., Martinez-Montes, E., Valdes-Sosa, P. A., Nishiyama, N., Mizuhara, H., & Yamaguchi, Y. (2004). Decomposing EEG data into space-time-frequency components using parallel factor analysis. *NeuroImage*, *22*(3), 1035–1045. doi: 10.1016/j.neuroimage.2004.03.039.

Mocks, J. (1988a). Topographic components model for event-related potentials and some biophysical considerations. *IEEE Transactions on Biomedical Engineering*, *35*, 482–484.

Mocks, J. (1988b). Decomposing event-related potentials: A new topographic components model. *Biological Psychology*, *26*, 199–215.

Morup, M. & Hansen, L. K. (2009). Automatic relevance determination for multiway models. *Journal of Chemometrics*, *23*, 352–363.

Morup, M., Hansen, L. K., & Arnfred, S. M. (2007). ERPWAVELAB a toolbox for multi-channel analysis of time-frequency transformed event related potentials. *Journal of Neuroscience Methods*, *161*(2), 361–368. doi: 10.1016/j.jneumeth.2006. 11.008.

Morup, M., Hansen, L. K., Herrmann, C. S., Parnas, J., & Arnfred, S. M. (2006). Parallel factor analysis as an exploratory tool for wavelet transformed event-related EEG. *NeuroImage*, *29*(3), 938–947. doi: 10.1016/j.neuroimage.2005.08.005.

Phan, A. H. & Cichocki, A. (2010). Tensor decomposition for feature extraction and classification problem. *IEICE Transactions on Fundamentals of Electronics, Communications and Computer Sciences*, *1*(1), 37–68.

Phan, A. H. & Cichocki, A. (2011). Extended HALS algorithm for nonnegative Tucker decomposition and its applications for multiway analysis and classification. *Neuro-computing*, *74*(11), 1956–1969.

Ramos-Loyo, J., Gonzalez-Garrido, A. A., Sanchez-Loyo, L. M., Medina, V., & Basar-Eroglu, C. (2009). Event-related potentials and event-related oscillations during identity and facial emotional processing in schizophrenia. *International Journal of Psychophysiology: Official Journal of the International Organization of Psychophysiology*, *71*(1), 84–90. doi: 10.1016/j.ijpsycho.2008.07.008.

Sidiropoulos, N. D. & Bro, R. (2000). On the uniqueness of multilinear decomposition of N-way arrays. *Journal of Chemometrics*, *14*, 229–239.

Smilde, A., Bro, R., & Geladi, P. (2004). *Multi-Way Analysis with Applications in the Chemical Sciences*. Wiley.

Stefanics, G., Haden, G., Huotilainen, M., Balazs, L., Sziller, I., Beke, A., . . . Winkler, I. (2007). Auditory temporal grouping in newborn infants. *Psychophysiology*, *44*(5), 697–702. doi: 10.1111/j.1469-8986.2007.00540.x.

Tallon-Baudry, C., Bertrand, O., Delpuech, C., & Pernier, J. (1996). Stimulus specificity of phase-locked and non-phase-locked 40 Hz visual responses in human. *The Journal of Neuroscience: The Official Journal of the Society for Neuroscience*, *16*(13), 4240–4249.

Tan, D. S. & Nijholt, A. (2010). *Brain–Computer Interfaces: Applying our Minds to Human–Computer Interaction*. London: Springer.

Timmerman, M. E. & Kiers, H. A. (2000). Three-mode principal components analysis: Choosing the numbers of components and sensitivity to local optima. *The British Journal of Mathematical and Statistical Psychology*, *53*(Pt 1), 1–16.

Tucker, L. R. (1966). Some mathematical notes on three-mode factor analysis. *Psychometrika*, *31*(3), 279–311.

Vanderperren, K., Mijovic, B., Novitskiy, N., Vanrumste, B., Stiers, P., Van den Bergh, B. R., . . . De Vos, M. (2013). Single trial ERP reading based on parallel factor analysis. *Psychophysiology*, *50*(1), 97–110. doi: 10.1111/j.1469-8986.2012.01405.x.

Wang, K., Begleiter, H., & Porjesz, B. (2000). Trilinear modeling of event-related potentials. *Brain Topography*, *12*, 263–271.

Yener, G. G., Guntekin, B., Oniz, A., & Basar, E. (2007). Increased frontal phase-locking of event-related theta oscillations in Alzheimer patients treated with cholinesterase inhibitors. *International Journal of Psychophysiology: Official Journal of the International Organization of Psychophysiology*, *64*(1), 46–52. doi: 10.1016/j.ijpsycho.2006.07.006.

Zhao, Q., Caiafa, C. F., Mandic, D. P., Zhang, L., Ball, T., Schulze-Bonhage, A., & Cichocki, A. (2011). Multilinear subspace regression: An orthogonal tensor decomposition approach. *Advances in Neural Information Processing Systems*, *24*, 1269–1277.

Zhou, G. & Cichocki, A. (2012). Fast and unique Tucker decompositions via multiway blind source separation. *Bulletin of the Polish Academy of Sciences-Technical Sciences*, *60*(3), 389405.

Zhou, G., Cichocki, A., & Xie, S. (2012). Fast nonnegative matrix/tensor factorization based on low-rank approximation. *IEEE Transactions on Signal Processing*, *60*(6), 2928–2940.

Chapter 5

Analysis of Ongoing EEG by NTF During Real-World Music Experiences

In the previous chapters in this book, the event-related potential (ERP) data are the object for data processing. The ERPs are elicited by controlled stimuli, which hardly occur in real-world experiences. In this chapter, we show how to analyze the ongoing electroencephalography (EEG) elicited by a naturalistic music stimulus.

5.1 Motivation

To decode the brain activity during real-world experiences, Hasson and his colleagues first reported their study using functional magnetic resonance imaging (fMRI) when the participants watched films in a scanner (Hasson, Nir, Levy, Fuhrmann, & Malach, 2004). They found similar responses among the participants. Subsequently, research in terms of ongoing brain activity during real-world experiences using naturalistic stimuli in both visual (Spiers & Maguire, 2007) and auditory modalities (Alluri *et al.*, 2012, 2013; Toiviainen, Alluri, Brattico, Wallentin, & Vuust, 2013) has attracted much interest. Today, studies on brain activity during real-world experiences are mostly conducted in terms of fMRI. In the Web of Science, when both "fMRI" and "real-world" are used as keywords in searching for articles, 198 papers were found in March 2014. However, in contrast to the fMRI studies, not as many papers are available that report relevant research using magnetoencephalography (MEG) (Campi, Parkkonen, Hari,

& Hyvarinen, 2013; Ding & Simon, 2012a, b; Hyvarinen, Ramkumar, Parkkonen, & Hari, 2010; Koskinen *et al.*, 2013; Ramkumar, Parkkonen, Hari, & Hyvarinen, 2012) or EEG (Cong *et al.*, 2012, 2013; Hadjidimitriou & Hadjileontiadis, 2012; Lin *et al.*, 2010; Lin, Duann, Feng, Chen, & Jung, 2014; Lu *et al.*, 2012; Mikutta, Altorfer, Strik, & Koenig, 2012; Wu, Li, & Yao, 2009; Wu, Li, & Yao, 2013).

The cost of fMRI and MEG has been known to be immense, which an ordinary brain imaging laboratory cannot afford. Therefore, studying brain activity during real-world experiences using EEG is very important. However, EEG data tend to be noisier, and studies on how to extract the brain activity elicited by the naturalistic stimulus are rare except for two recent papers (Cong *et al.*, 2013; Lin *et al.*, 2014). In these two papers, independent component analysis (ICA) was applied, and the temporal course of an EEG oscillation was correlated with the temporal course of a musical feature of the music stimulus. When the correlation coefficient was significantly large, the corresponding component was regarded as elicited by the naturalistic music.

To obtain the temporal course of an EEG oscillation, the spectrogram of an independent component is calculated (Cong *et al.*, 2013; Lin *et al.*, 2014). The spectrogram is actually the absolute value of the short-time Fourier transform. On the basis of this characteristic, when the spectrogram of the EEG data in the electrode field is obtained, the EEG data of a subject can be represented by a third-order tensor (three-way data array; please see Figure 4.2). Consequently, applying the nonnegative tensor factorization (NTF) to decompose this tensor would be very natural (please see Figure 4.3). In a previous study, a fourth-order ongoing EEG tensor of the spectrograms of 14 subjects was decomposed by NTF (Cong *et al.*, 2012). In this chapter, we show how the third-order ongoing EEG tensor of the spectrogram of a subject can be analyzed.

5.2 Third-Order Ongoing EEG Tensor of a Spectrogram

The EEG data of a right-handed and healthy adult in Finland are used in this study. The participant was not a music expert. An entire musical piece of modern tango — Astor Piazzolla — was used as test stimulus. The 8.5-min Piazzolla tango was recorded in a concert in Lausanne, Switzerland

(Alluri *et al.*, 2012). During the experiment, the participant was asked to open his eyes and attentively listen to the music.

The EEG data were recorded using a 10–20 system with BioSemi bioactive electrode caps (64 electrodes in the cap plus 5 external electrodes at the tip of the nose, left and right mastoids, and both horizontally and vertically around the right eye). The sampling rate was 2048 Hz, and the EEG data were saved for offline processing. The external electrode at the nose was used as reference, and the data were preprocessed in EEGLAB (Delorme & Makeig, 2004), downsampled to 256 Hz, and high-pass (HP) and low-pass (LP) filtered using 1- and 30-Hz cutoff frequencies, respectively. ICA was applied to remove the eye blinks (Cong *et al.*, 2013).

After the preprocessing, short-time Fourier transform was applied on the ongoing EEG data of each channel to obtain the spectrogram of the data. The duration of the sliding window was 3 s, and the overlap between two segments was 2 s. The duration and the overlap were chosen in terms of the musical feature extraction (presented in the next section). Then, the third-order ongoing EEG tensor of the spectrogram was produced. The sizes of the tensor here were 146 (frequency bins, 1–30 Hz) × 510 s × 64 channels.

Figure 5.1 shows the spectrogram of the ongoing EEG at the typical electrode locations along the scalp. Evidently, strong oscillations exist between 5 and 10 Hz.

5.3 Musical Features of the Naturalistic Music

Five musical (tonal and rhythmic) features were used here, which were studied in previous papers (Alluri *et al.*, 2012; Cong *et al.*, 2013). To extract the features, the 512-s-long music was first segmented into 510 frames using a sliding rectangular window. The frame duration was 3 s, and the overlap between two adjacent frames was 2 s. The features in each frame were then extracted. Next, five temporal courses of these features were produced under a sampling frequency of 1 Hz. The details of the feature extraction can be found in previous studies (Alluri *et al.*, 2012; Lartillot & Toiviainen, 2007). Figure 5.2 shows the temporal courses of the five musical features. We note that the temporal courses of the musical

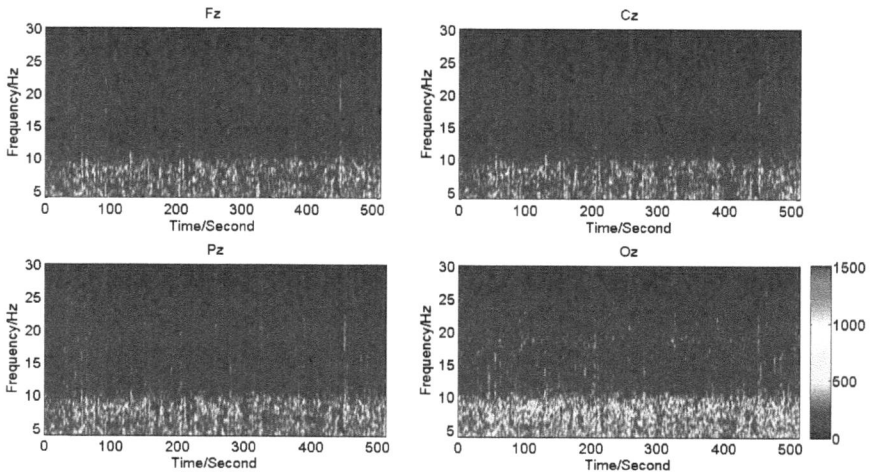

Figure 5.1   Spectrogram of ongoing EEG at four typical locations along the scalp.

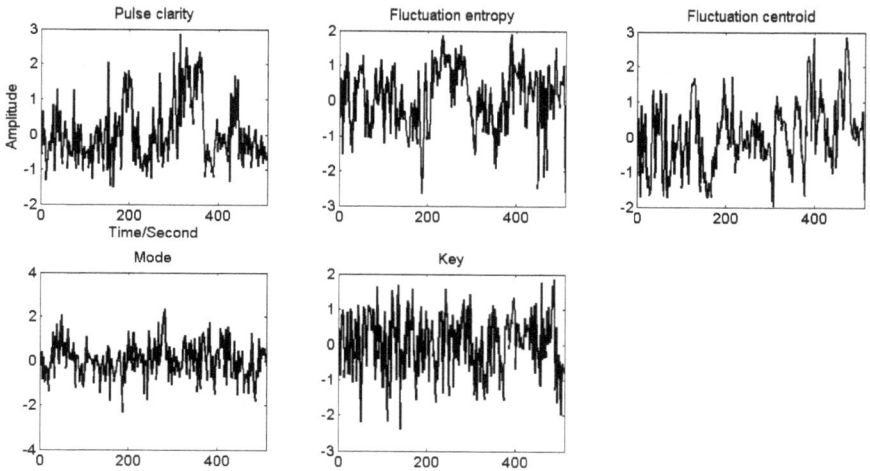

Figure 5.2   Five long-term musical features. The musical features are denoted as "#1: Pulse clarity," "#2: Fluctuation entropy," "#3: Fluctuation centroid," "#4: Mode," and "#5: Key" [adapted from Alluri *et al.* (2012) and Cong *et al.* (2013)].

features were not significantly correlated with the temporal courses of the alpha or theta oscillations shown in Figure 5.1 (Cong *et al.*, 2013).

5.4 NTF on the Spectrogram of Ongoing EEG

We use the nonnegative canonical polyadic decomposition (NCPD) (please see Chapter 4) to decompose the third-order ongoing EEG tensor of the spectrogram. We determine the number of components on the basis of the criterion of the explained variance. The threshold is set to 95%. For this purpose, the time and space modes are merged, and the third-order tensor is then reshaped into a matrix with a size of 146 by 32,640. Figure 5.3 shows the eigenvalues of the sample covariance matrix of the tensor-reshaped matrix. In terms of the 95% threshold, "31" is chosen as the number of extracted components for the NCPD on the third-order ongoing EEG tensor. Then, the low-rank approximation (LRA)-based NCPD (Cong *et al.*, 2014) is applied on the third-order tensor to extract 31 temporal, 31 spectral, and 31 spatial components. We should note that the order or the variance of the components in any mode is not determined. After the algorithm converges, the fit of the 31-component model is 71% relative to norm-1 in Eq. (4-7) (i.e., absolute value).

Subsequently, the 31 temporal components and the five musical features are correlated with one another. The threshold used to determine the significance of the correlation coefficient is based on permutation and Monte Carlo simulations (Alluri *et al.*, 2012; Cong *et al.*, 2013; Groppe, Urbach, & Kutas, 2011). We use fair level at $P = 0.05$ for the threshold. Then, six temporal components are selected. Meanwhile, the corresponding spectral and spatial components are chosen. The rationale for the selection is shown in Figure 4.3. Furthermore, the reliable spatial component is not scattered but dipolar (Cong *et al.*, 2013; Delorme, Palmer, Onton, Oostenveld, & Makeig, 2012; Lin *et al.*, 2014). On the basis of this criterion, two spatial components are rejected. Finally, four among the 31 components are chosen to be regarded as the reliable brain activities elicited by the naturalistic music stimulus. They are shown in Figure 5.4.

(a)

(b)

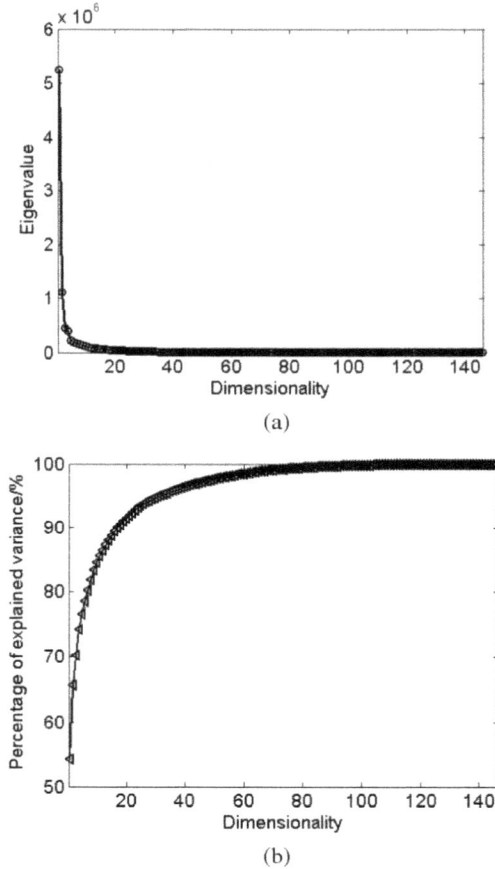

Figure 5.3   (a) Eigenvalues and (b) Explained variance of the cumulated eigenvalues.

Among the five musical features, four are found to significantly correlate with the temporal components extracted by the NCPD. Among the four spatial components, three components show the posterior alpha, and one component shows the central and frontal alpha. This result is consistent with the previous findings that used the ICA (Cong *et al.*, 2013; Lin *et al.*, 2014). With the application of the NCPD on the third-order ongoing EEG tensor of the spectrogram, calculating the EEG oscillation is not necessary, which is required when ICA is used (Cong *et al.*, 2013). Consequently, examining the spectral property of the EEG using tensor decomposition would be more objective.

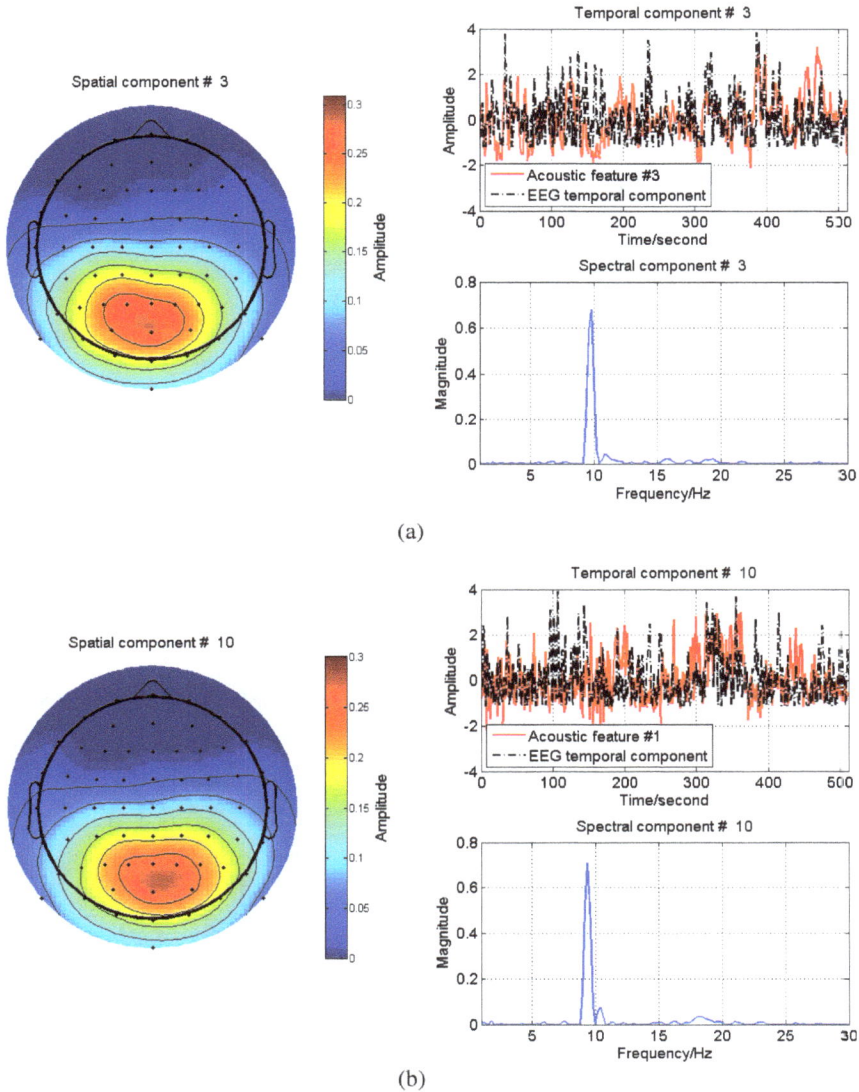

(a)

(b)

Figure 5.4 Selected components extracted by the NCPD on the third-order ongoing EEG tensor of the spectrogram. The temporal components are significantly correlated with the musical features ($P < 0.05$). The spatial components are dipolar. Each temporal component is standardized, i.e., the mean is zero, and the variance is one.

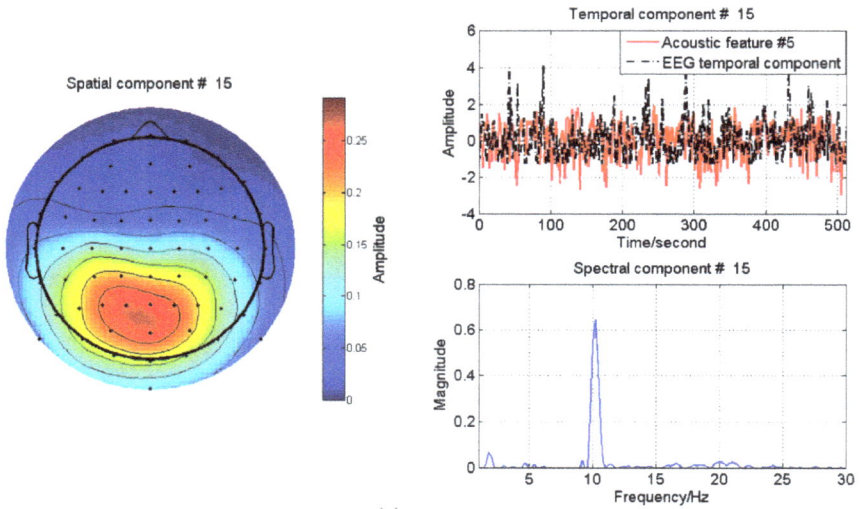

(c)

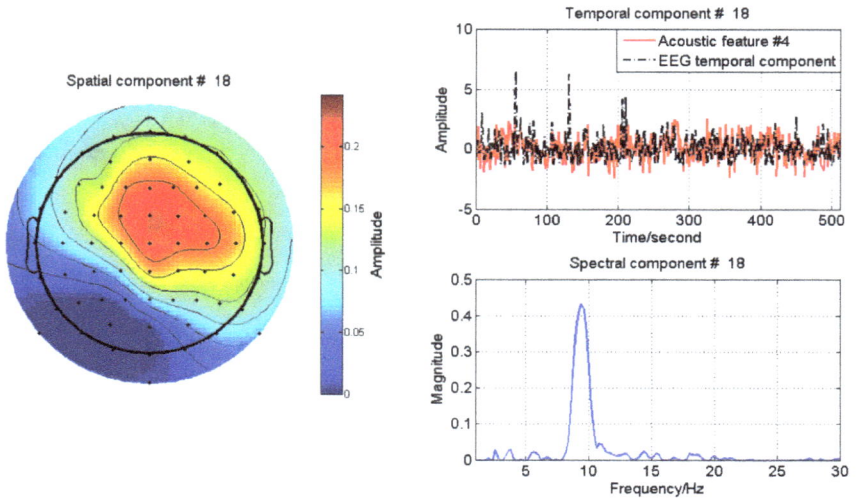

(d)

Figure 5.4   *Continued.*

5.5 Summary

With the application of the NTF in terms of the CP model on the third-order ongoing EEG tensor of the spectrogram, we have determined the reliable brain activities when a participant listens to a naturalistic music. The EEG tensor was simultaneously filtered by the NTF in the time, frequency, and space domains.

5.6 Existing Problem and Solution

In the ICA, the variance and polarity of an independent component are indeterminate, and they can be theoretically completely corrected (Cong, Kalyakin, & Ristaniemi, 2011; Cong, Kalyakin, Zheng, & Ristaniemi, 2011). The variance and polarity of a component extracted by the NTF in any mode are also inherently indeterminate. In theory, correcting the indeterminacies using the NTF is not currently possible. Therefore, the NTF can be appropriately used only to analyze the data of a subject in order to examine the pattern of the brain activity of interest. To investigate the variance in the brain activity, NTF must be performed on the group-level ongoing EEG data, which can be a third- or fourth-order tensor.

References

Alluri, V., Toiviainen, P., Jaaskelainen, I. P., Glerean, E., Sams, M., & Brattico, E. (2012). Large-scale brain networks emerge from dynamic processing of musical timbre, key and rhythm. *NeuroImage*, *59*, 3677–3689. doi: 10.1016/j.neuroimage.2011.11.019.

Alluri, V., Toiviainen, P., Lund, T. E., Wallentin, M., Vuust, P., Nandi, A. K., . . . Brattico, E. (2013). From Vivaldi to Beatles and back: Predicting lateralized brain responses to music. *NeuroImage*, *83*, 627–636. doi: 10.1016/j.neuroimage.2013.06.064.

Campi, C., Parkkonen, L., Hari, R., & Hyvarinen, A. (2013). Non-linear canonical correlation for joint analysis of MEG signals from two subjects. *Frontiers in Neuroscience*, *7*, 107. doi: 10.3389/fnins.2013.00107.

Cong, F., Alluri, V., Nandi, A. K., Toiviainen, P., Fa, R., Abu-Jamous, B., . . . Ristaniemi, T. (2013). Linking brain responses to naturalistic music through analysis of ongoing EEG and stimulus features. *IEEE Transactions on Multimedia*, *15*(5), 1060–1069.

Cong, F., Kalyakin, I., & Ristaniemi, T. (2011). Can back-projection fully resolve polarity indeterminacy of ICA in study of ERP? *Biomedical Signal Processing and Control*, *6*(4), 422–426.

Cong, F., Kalyakin, I., Zheng, C., & Ristaniemi, T. (2011). Analysis on subtracting projection of extracted independent components from EEG recordings. *Biomedizinische Technik/ Biomedical Engineering*, *56*(4), 223–234.

Cong, F., Phan, A. H., Zhao, Q., Nandi, A. K., Alluri, V., Toiviainen, P., . . . Ristaniemi, T. (2012). Analysis of Ongoing EEG Elicited by Natural Music Stimuli Using Nonnegative Tensor Factorization. *Proceeding of the 2012 European Signal Processing Conference (EUSIPCO-2012)*, Bucharest, Romania, August 27–31, Bucharest, Romania, 494–498.

Cong, F., Zhou, G., Astikainen, P., Zhao, Q., Wu, Q., Nandi, A.K., . . . Cichocki, A. (2014). Low-rank approximation based nonnegative multi-way array decomposition on event-related potentials. *International Journal of Neural Systems*. doi: 10.1142/S012906571440005X.

Delorme, A. & Makeig, S. (2004). EEGLAB: An open source toolbox for analysis of single-trial EEG dynamics including independent component analysis. *Journal of Neuroscience Methods*, *134*(1), 9–21. doi: 10.1016/j.jneumeth.2003.10.009.

Delorme, A., Palmer, J., Onton, J., Oostenveld, R., & Makeig, S. (2012). Independent EEG sources are dipolar. *PloS One*, *7*(2), e30135. doi: 10.1371/journal.pone.0030135.

Ding, N. & Simon, J. Z. (2012a). Emergence of neural encoding of auditory objects while listening to competing speakers. *Proceedings of the National Academy of Sciences of the United States of America*, *109*(29), 11854–11859. doi: 10.1073/pnas.1205381109; 10.1073/pnas.1205381109.

Ding, N. & Simon, J. Z. (2012b). Neural coding of continuous speech in auditory cortex during monaural and dichotic listening. *Journal of Neurophysiology*, *107*(1), 78–89. doi: 10.1152/jn.00297.2011.

Groppe, D. M., Urbach, T. P., & Kutas, M. (2011). Mass univariate analysis of event-related brain potentials/fields I: A critical tutorial review. *Psychophysiology*, *48*(12), 1711–1725. doi: 10.1111/j.1469-8986.2011.01273.x.

Hadjidimitriou, S. K. & Hadjileontiadis, L. J. (2012). Toward an EEG-based recognition of music liking using time-frequency analysis. *IEEE Transactions on Bio-medical Engineering*, *59*(12), 3498–3510. doi: 10.1109/TBME.2012.2217495.

Hasson, U., Nir, Y., Levy, I., Fuhrmann, G., & Malach, R. (2004). Intersubject synchronization of cortical activity during natural vision. *Science (New York, N.Y.)*, *303*(5664), 1634–1640. doi: 10.1126/science.1089506.

Hyvarinen, A., Ramkumar, P., Parkkonen, L., & Hari, R. (2010). Independent component analysis of short-time Fourier transforms for spontaneous EEG/MEG analysis. *NeuroImage*, *49*(1), 257–271. doi: 10.1016/j.neuroimage.2009.08.028.

Koskinen, M., Viinikanoja, J., Kurimo, M., Klami, A., Kaski, S., & Hari, R. (2013). Identifying fragments of natural speech from the listener's MEG signals. *Human Brain Mapping*, *34*(6), 1477–1489. doi: 10.1002/hbm.22004.

Lartillot, O. & Toiviainen, P. (2007). MIR in Matlab (II): A toolbox for musical feature extraction from audio. Paper presented at the *Proceeding of International Conference on Music Information Retrieval 2007*.

Lin, Y. P., Wang, C. H., Jung, T. P., Wu, T. L., Jeng, S. K., Duann, J. R., & Chen, J. H. (2010). EEG-based emotion recognition in music listening. *IEEE Transactions on Bio-Medical Engineering*, *57*(7), 1798–1806. doi: 10.1109/TBME.2010.2048568.

Lin, Y. P., Duann, J. R., Feng, W. F., Chen, J. H., & Jung, T. P. (2014). Revealing spatio-spectral electroencephalographic dynamics of musical mode and tempo perception by independent component analysis. *Journal of NeuroEngineering and Rehabilitation*, *11*(18), 1–11.

Lu, J., Wu, D., Yang, H., Luo, C., Li, C., & Yao, D. (2012). Scale-free brain-wave music from simultaneously EEG and fMRI recordings. *PloS One*, *7*(11), e49773. doi: 10.1371/journal.pone.0049773.

Mikutta, C., Altorfer, A., Strik, W., & Koenig, T. (2012). Emotions, arousal, and frontal alpha rhythm asymmetry during Beethoven's 5th symphony. *Brain Topography*, *25*(4), 423–430. doi: 10.1007/s10548-012-0227-0.

Ramkumar, P., Parkkonen, L., Hari, R., & Hyvarinen, A. (2012). Characterization of neuromagnetic brain rhythms over time scales of minutes using spatial independent component analysis. *Human Brain Mapping*, *33*(7), 1648–1662. doi: 10.1002/hbm.21303.

Spiers, H. J. & Maguire, E. A. (2007). Decoding human brain activity during real-world experiences. *Trends in Cognitive Sciences*, *11*(8), 356–365. doi: 10.1016/j.tics.2007.06.002.

Toiviainen, P., Alluri, V., Brattico, E., Wallentin, M., & Vuust, P. (2013). Capturing the musical brain with Lasso: Dynamic decoding of musical features from fMRI data. *NeuroImage*, *88C*, 170–180. doi: 10.1016/j.neuroimage.2013.11.017.

Wu, D., Li, C. Y., & Yao, D. Z. (2009). Scale-free music of the brain. *PloS One*, *4*(6), e5915. doi: 10.1371/journal.pone.0005915.

Wu, D., Li, C., & Yao, D. (2013). Scale-free brain quartet: Artistic filtering of multi-channel brainwave music. *PloS One*, *8*(5), e64046. doi: 10.1371/journal.pone.0064046.

Appendix

Introduction to Basic Knowledge of Mismatch Negativity

In this appendix, we introduce the history of mismatch negativity (MMN), the paradigm to elicit MMN, the corresponding knowledge of MMN and its temporal, spectral, time-frequency, and spatial properties. Most of the contents are based on Fengyu Cong's dissertation in Finland (Cong, 2010).

A.1 Brief History of MMN

MMN was first reported in 1978 (Näätänen, Gaillard, & Mäntysalo, 1978). These authors described MMN as a "physiological mismatch process caused by a sensory input deviating from the memory trace ('template') formed by a frequent 'background' stimulus (p. 324)". Moreover, MMN can be attention free, i.e., to generate MMN a participant does not necessarily pay attention to the stimulus paradigm; its amplitude is very small, and usually is up to several micro volts with a peak latency of 100–200 ms (Näätänen et al., 2012; Näätänen, Kujala, Kreegipuu, et al., 2011; Näätänen, Kujala, & Winkler, 2011).

Since MMN was isolated in 1978, dozens of research groups all over the world have been studying MMN. The society of interest in MMN has grown extensively over the past three decades. Among all ERPs, only for MMN there is a special international conference focused on MMN research and clinical applications. Six congresses focused on MMN have already been held. These include: first in Finland (1998), second in Spain (2000), third in France (2003), fourth in the United Kingdom (2006), fifth in Hungary (2009), and the sixth took place in New York, USA in 2012. Nowadays, hundreds of researchers from all over the world participate in the

MMN conference. Over 1000 journal papers have been published in various scientific journals as reporting the study of MMN. Without doubt, MMN has become an important stream in research of cognitive neuroscience, clinical neuroscience, and applications (Näätänen *et al.*, 2012; Näätänen, Kujala, Kreegipuu, *et al.*, 2011; Näätänen, Kujala, & Winkler, 2011).

A.2 Paradigm to Elicit MMN

Today, it is well known that MMN can be elicited through an oddball paradigm and it is usually observed from difference wave. Under this elicitation procedure, MMN has been interpreted through the memory-based model (Näätänen, 2001), the regularity-violation model (Winkler, 2007), and the adaptation model (May & Tiitinen, 2010). This book obeys the first model and it is illustrated in Figure A.1.

For example, several consecutive standard stimuli make the brain formulate the sensory memory and then the incoming deviant stimulus is slightly different from information in the formed memory. And then, brain will implement a comparison process. In such scenario, MMN can be generated. For the auditory stimulus, the deviant type can be the duration, the intensity, the frequency, the location, and so on (Näätänen *et al.*, 2012; Näätänen, Kujala, Kreegipuu, *et al.*, 2011; Näätänen, Kujala, & Winkler, 2011). For the visual stimulus, it can be emotions and orientations (Astikainen, Cong, Ristaniemi, & Hietanen, 2013; Astikainen & Hietanen, 2009; Astikainen, Lillstrang, & Ruusuvirta, 2008).

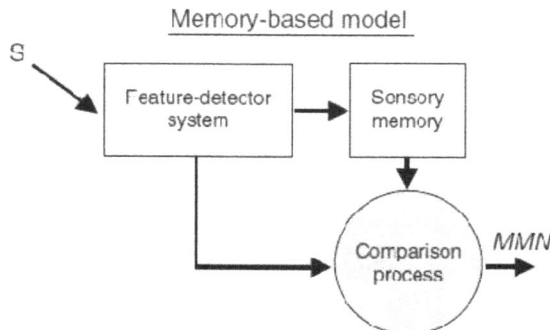

Figure A.1   Memory-based MMN Model [adapted from May & Tiitinen (2009)].

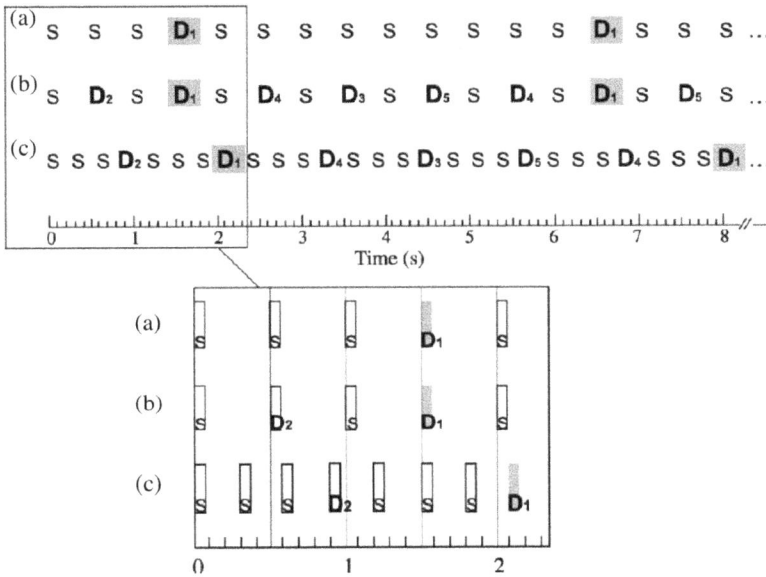

Figure A.2   Oddball, optimum-1, and optimum-2 paradigms [adapted from Näätänen, Pakarinen, Rinne, & Takegata (2004)].

Typically, an oddball paradigm to elicit MMN includes two concepts about the duration. One is an inter-stimulus-interval (ISI) and the other is a stimulus-onset-asynchrony (SOA). ISI is the duration of a silent gap between two adjacent stimuli. SOA is the time period from the onset of one stimulus to the onset of the next stimulus.

The conventional oddball paradigm is frequently used in the study of MMN. It is illustrated in Figure A.2(a) (Näätänen, Pakarinen, Rinne, & Takegata, 2004). However, one main disadvantage of this type of paradigm is time-consuming. It often takes hours to achieve well-structured MMN from one subject, which is not suitable for young children and clinical populations (Näätänen *et al.*, 2004; Pakarinen, Takegata, Rinne, Huotilainen, & Näätänen, 2007). Thus, Professor Näätänen and colleagues invented the optimum-1 and optimum-2 paradigms, consisting of five different deviants (Näätänen *et al.*, 2004). Figure A.2 demonstrates these deviants. SOA and ISI for (a) and (b) are 500 ms and 425 ms, and for (c) are 300 ms and 225 ms. Näätänen and colleagues (2004) declared that both the optimum-1 and optimum-2 could effectively elicit MMN and the new procedures significantly saved much time. In short, to achieve five MMNs under five deviants, the time taken by the conventional oddball paradigm is five times that (15 mins in Näätänen *et al.*, 2004) taken by the optimum-1 procedure.

Meanwhile, it was reported that the optimum-2 paradigm produced smaller MMN peak amplitude (Näätänen *et al.*, 2004). Indeed, under optimum-2, ISI is shorter and standard stimuli are more repeated in contrast to the conventional oddball and optimum-1 paradigms. Thus, such a result reported by Näätänen and colleagues (2004) may conflict with common knowledge in eliciting MMN, i.e., the shorter ISI and more standard stimuli may correspond to a larger MMN peak amplitude (Näätänen *et al.*, 2012). Nevertheless, Professor Erich Schroger stated that longer ISI could contribute MMN with larger peak amplitudes under the frequency deviant (Schroger, 1996). By now, no solid illustrations for such conflicts have been made.

Another way to obtain fast recordings is through uninterrupted sound, i.e., the ISI is zero. In 1995, Dr. Elina Pihko and colleagues used such a continuous sound to elicit MMN for the investigation of people's ability to detect temporal changes (Pihko, Leppasaari, & Lyytinen, 1995). Recently, the same paradigm has also been used in the MMN study of typically developing children, children with reading disabilities (RD) and children with attention deficit hyperactivity disorders (ADHD) (Huttunen-Scott, Kaartinen, Tolvanen, & Lyytinen, 2008; Huttunen, Halonen, Kaartinen, & Lyytinen, 2007; Kalyakin, Gonzalez, Ivannikov, & Lyytinen, 2009; Kalyakin *et al.*, 2007; Kalyakin, Gonzalez, Kärkkäinen, & Lyytinen, 2008). This took approximately only 15 min to collect 700 trials and thus is very promising in the application to young children and clinical groups. As a result, this study also adopts such a continuous sound procedure. Figure A.3 illustrates this paradigm. The uninterrupted sound has alternating 100 ms sine tones of 600 Hz and 800 Hz (repeated stimuli). There is no pause between the alternating tones and their amplitudes do not change. During the experiment, 15% of the 600 Hz tones are randomly replaced by shorter tones of 50 ms and 30 ms duration (called as dev50 and dev30). The deviants consist of 7.5% of 50 ms deviants and 7.5% 30 ms deviants. There are at least six repetitions of the alternating 100 ms tones between deviants.

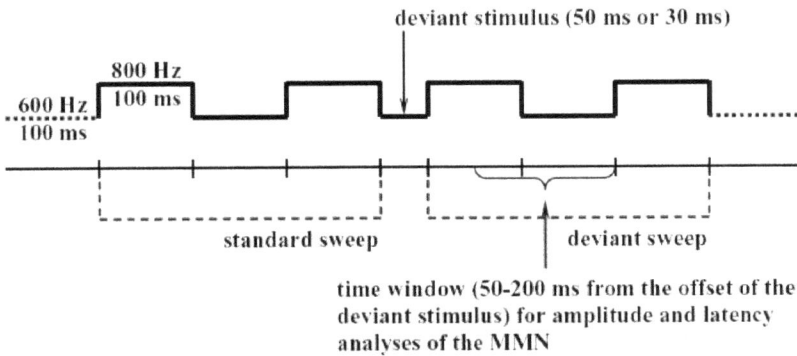

deviant stimulus (50 ms or 30 ms)

800 Hz
100 ms

.600 Hz.
100 ms

standard sweep   deviant sweep

time window (50-200 ms from the offset of the
deviant stimulus) for amplitude and latency
analyses of the MMN

Figure A.3   A schematic illustration of the stimulus sequence to elicit MMN through the
continuous sound [adapted from Kalyakin et al. (2007)].

A.3 Basic Psychological Knowledge of MMN

As mentioned earlier, MMN can be elicited through the oddball paradigm
(Näätänen *et al.*, 2012; Näätänen, Kujala, Kreegipuu, *et al.*, 2011). For
example, one oddball sequence could be "S S S S D1 S S S D2 S S S S S
D3 S S S...", where "S" denotes the standard stimulus, i.e., the repeated
stimulus, and "D1", "D2", or "D3" represents the deviant stimulus of the
same type. The three deviants have different magnitudes of the deviance to
the standard stimulus. MMN has such a property: the larger is the magnitude
of the deviance, the larger is the peak amplitude and the shorter is the peak
latency of the MMN (Näätänen *et al.*, 2012; Näätänen, Kujala, Kreegipuu,
et al., 2011). This is the basic psychological knowledge of MMN.

Indeed, although it is impossible to localize the true MMN sources,
the MMN functions have been somewhat unveiled (Näätänen *et al.*, 2012;
Näätänen, Kujala, Kreegipuu, *et al.*, 2011). Meanwhile, as suggested by
Dr. Vigario and Professor Oja (Vigario & Oja, 2008), the evaluation of the
ERP processing should be based on the knowledge of ERPs by the expert.
Thus, the criteria used to estimate the success to extract MMN should be
based on the analysis of psychological knowledge and properties of MMN.

A.4 Properties of MMN

In the single channel EEG recordings, MMN has its own temporal, spectral,
and time-frequency features, and from the multichannel, the spatial features

between the MMN source and EEG recordings can be exploited. They are introduced as follows.

A.4.1 *Temporal property*

ERPs are time-locked according to its elicitation paradigm (Luck, 2005), which contributes its temporal feature. For example, as illustrated in Figure A.3, an MMN peak may appear in the time frame between 50 and 200 ms after the offset of the deviant stimulus (Pihko *et al.*, 1995). Out of that frame, no MMN can be observed. So, the temporal feature is derived from the paradigm to elicit MMN and a time frame within which the MMN peak may appear should be defined to describe its temporal feature.

A.4.2 *Spectral property*

The spectral feature of MMN includes two parts. One is the frequency range of MMN and the other is the spectral structure within that frequency range.

Since the digital filter was applied to filter out the interference, the frequency range of MMN has been attractive to researchers. Different frequency bands have been used to remove the interference from the averaged MMN trace. For example, Kalyakin *et al.* (2007) made a deep analysis on the cutoff frequencies for the MMN frequency band of children and concluded that the optimal MMN frequency band of children was 2–8.5 Hz under an uninterrupted sound paradigm; Stefanics G. *et al.* (Stefanics *et al.*, 2007, 2009; adopted the 2.5–16 Hz and 1.5–16 Hz to achieve MMN of neonates respectively; for visual inspection of MMN, Sinkkonen and Tervaniemi (2000) recommended a 1–20 Hz band; Tervaniemi *et al.* (1999) had always used 2–10 Hz band-pass digital filter for subsequently analyzing MMN peak amplitude and latency; Sabri and Campbell (2002) set the band of MMN as 3–12 Hz. In summary, the frequency of MMN is very low. Most of the studies simply reported that a certain frequency band was used for MMN. This is not convincing for the further application by other researchers. In order to determine the frequency band of MMN, Kalyakin *et al.* (2007) designed a special paradigm. It is repeated in this study. This method consists of two groups of digital filters. One is the group of low-pass filters to seek the high cutoff frequency and the other is the group of high-pass filters to isolate the low cutoff frequency. For example, when the high cutoff frequency of the low-pass filter gradually reduces, the peak amplitude of MMN can be measured at every high cutoff frequency. Then, the change of the peak amplitudes may be discovered along the change of the high cutoff frequencies. The frequency with the largest MMN peak amplitude can be considered as the high bound of the MMN frequency range. The low bound of the MMN frequency range can also be found this way. For details, see Kalyakin *et al.* (2007). Since the data set used in this study is identical to that used by Kalyakin *et al.* (2007), 2–8.5 Hz is used as the optimal frequency band of MMN hereinafter. For other studies, the frequency band may be determined by the procedure mentioned above.

Another point is to determine the spectral structure within a frequency band. For example, the frequency corresponding to the most powerful energy is a critical parameter within the frequency range of MMN. This has not been well discussed in previous publications. Picton *et al.* (Picton, Alain, Otten, Ritter, & Achim, 2000) considered that most of the MMN's energy lay in the 2–5 Hz frequency range. Consequently, in this book, the power of the frequency is regarded to peak around 5 Hz.

A.4.3 *Time-frequency property*

Frequency analysis of ERPs is very important. However, the same spectral features in the frequency domain might correspond to different waveforms in the time domain. Thus, it is necessary to perform the time-frequency analysis. Figures A.3 and A.4 demonstrate the advantage in using the time-frequency feature to discriminate different signals. Figure A.4 depicts the waveforms of two signals and the spectrums of the two signals. Figure A.5 shows their time-frequency representation. As shown in Figures A.4 and A.5, the difference between the two signals is most evident under the time-frequency representation despite the similar waveforms and almost identical spectral structures that the two signals share. This is the advantage of the time-frequency analysis in discriminating different signals.

Specifically, the rectangle area in Figure A.5 determines the region of interest (ROI). The power in ROI of Figure A.5(A) is much larger than that

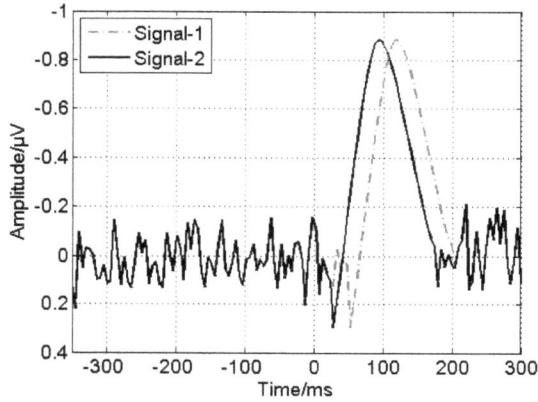

(a)

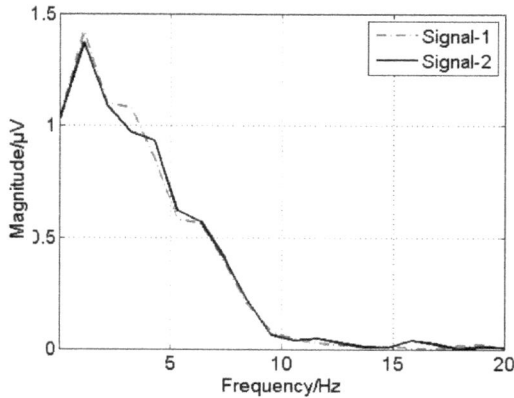

(b)

Figure A.4 (a) Waveform, (b) Spectrum.

of Figure A.5(B). In this case, the ROI is defined through the temporal and spectral features of MMN mentioned above. For example, the time frame of ROI is from 50 to 200 ms and the frequency range of ROI is from 2 to 8.5 Hz. These four numbers determine a rectangle.

When different signals have determinant variances, respectively, the values of ROIs among them are comparable. Subsequently, the time-frequency feature of MMN can be derived from the averaged power within ROI of the time-frequency representation. It is defined through the averaged power of all time-frequency points within the ROI. Therefore, such a

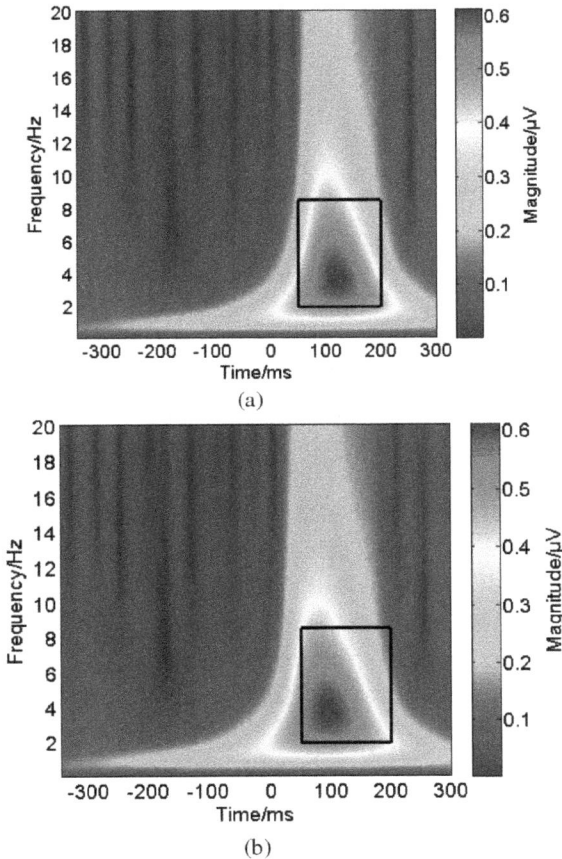

Figure A.5 (A) Time-frequency analysis of signal-1, (B) Time-frequency analysis of signal-2.

parameter can spontaneously reflect the temporal and spectral information of MMN.

A.4.4 *Topography*

The spatial information includes two parts: One is the topography of a certain ERP, and the other is the relationship between the brain sources and EEG recordings at the scalp. Every ERP has a certain distribution over the scalp. The distribution tends to include two aspects. Figure A.6 shows one example of auditory MMN's topography. For example, one is

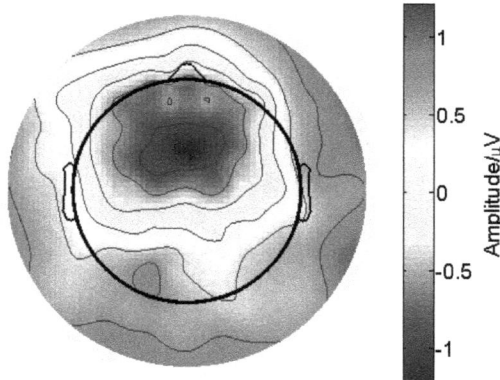

Figure A.6   One example of auditory MMN's topography.

related to the energy of the MMN peak amplitude and the other to the polarity of the MMN peak amplitude. These are the topographic features of an ERP. Particularly, MMN elicited by the auditory modality usually has relatively larger peak amplitude at the frontal area, and its polarity is negative at the frontal, central, and parietal area, and is positive at the mastoid under the reference to the tip of the nose (Näätänen *et al.*, 2012; Näätänen, Kujala, Kreegipuu, *et al.*, 2011). Such information is very critical to the determination of a proper MMN component.

References

Astikainen, P., Cong, F., Ristaniemi, T., & Hietanen, J. K. (2013). Event-related potentials to unattended changes in facial expressions: detection of regularity violations or encoding of emotions? *Frontiers in Human Neuroscience*, 7, 557. doi: 10.3389/fnhum.2013.00557.

Astikainen, P. & Hietanen, J. K. (2009). Event-related potentials to task-irrelevant changes in facial expressions. *Behavioral and Brain Functions: BBF*, 5, 30. doi: 10.1186/1744-9081-5-30.

Astikainen, P., Lillstrang, E., & Ruusuvirta, T. (2008). Visual mismatch negativity for changes in orientation–a sensory memory-dependent response. *The European Journal of Neuroscience*, 28(11), 2319–2324. doi: 10.1111/j.1460-9568.2008.06510.x.

Cong, F. (2010). *Evaluation and Extraction of Mismatch Negativity through Exploiting Temporal, Spectral, Time-frequency and Spatial Features.* (Ph.D.), University of Jyvaskyla, Jyvaskyla, Finland.

Huttunen-Scott, T., Kaartinen, J., Tolvanen, A., & Lyytinen, H. (2008). Mismatch negativity (MMN) elicited by duration deviations in children with reading disorder, attention deficit or both. *International Journal of Psychophysiology: Official*

Journal of the International Organization of Psychophysiology, 69(1), 69–77. doi: 10.1016/j.ijpsycho.2008.03.002.

Huttunen, T., Halonen, A., Kaartinen, J., & Lyytinen, H. (2007). Does mismatch negativity show differences in reading-disabled children compared to normal children and children with attention deficit? *Developmental Neuropsychology, 31*(3), 453–470. doi: 10.1080/87565640701229656.

Kalyakin, I., Gonzalez, M., Ivannikov, I., & Lyytinen, H. (2009). Extraction of the mismatch negativity elicited by sound duration decrements: A comparison of three procedures. *Data & Knowledge Engineering, 68*(12), 1411–1426.

Kalyakin, I., Gonzalez, N., Joutsensalo, J., Huttunen, T., Kaartinen, J., & Lyytinen, H. (2007). Optimal digital filtering versus difference waves on the mismatch negativity in an uninterrupted sound paradigm. *Developmental Neuropsychology, 31*(3), 429–452. doi: 10.1080/87565640701229607.

Kalyakin, I., Gonzalez, N., Kärkkäinen, T., & Lyytinen, H. (2008). Independent component analysis on the mismatch negativity in an uninterrupted sound paradigm. *Journal of Neuroscience Methods, 174*(2), 301–312. doi: 10.1016/j.jneumeth.2008. 07.012.

Luck, S. J. (2005). *An Introduction to the Event-Related Potential Technique.* Cambridge, MA: The MIT Press.

May, P. J. & Tiitinen, H. (2010). Mismatch negativity (MMN), the deviance-elicited auditory deflection, explained. *Psychophysiology, 47*(1), 66–122. doi: 10.1111/j. 1469-8986.2009.00856.x.

Näätänen, R. (2001). The perception of speech sounds by the human brain as reflected by the mismatch negativity (MMN) and its magnetic equivalent (MMNm). *Psychophysiology, 38*(1), 1–21.

Näätänen, R., Gaillard, A. W., & Mäntysalo, S. (1978). Early selective-attention effect on evoked potential reinterpreted. *Acta Psychologica, 42*(4), 313–329.

Näätänen, R., Kujala, T., Escera, C., Baldeweg, T., Kreegipuu, K., Carlson, C., & Ponton, C. (2012). The mismatch negativity (MMN) — A unique window to disturbed central auditory processing in ageing and different clinical conditions. *Clinical Neurophysiology: Official Journal of the International Federation of Clinical Neurophysiology, 123*, 424–458.

Näätänen, R., Kujala, T., Kreegipuu, K., Carlson, S., Escera, C., Baldeweg, T., & Pontor, C. (2011). The mismatch negativity: an index of cognitive decline in neuropsychiatric and neurological diseases and in ageing. *Brain: A Journal of Neurology, 134* (Pt 12), 3432–3450. doi: 10.1093/brain/awr064.

Näätänen, R., Kujala, T., & Winkler, I. (2011). Auditory processing that leads to conscious perception: a unique window to central auditory processing opened by the mismatch negativity and related responses. *Psychophysiology, 48*(1), 4–22. doi: 10.1111/j. 1469-8986.2010.01114.x.

Näätänen, R., Pakarinen, S., Rinne, T., & Takegata, R. (2004). The mismatch negativity (MMN): Towards the optimal paradigm. *Clinical Neurophysiology: Official Journal of the International Federation of Clinical Neurophysiology, 115*(1), 140–144.

Pakarinen, S., Takegata, R., Rinne, T., Huotilainen, M., & Näätänen, R. (2007). Measurement of extensive auditory discrimination profiles using the mismatch negativity (MMN) of the auditory event-related potential (ERP). *Clinical Neurophysiology: Official*

Journal of the International Federation of Clinical Neurophysiology, *118*(1), 177–185. doi: 10.1016/j.clinph.2006.09.001.

Picton, T. W., Alain, C., Otten, L., Ritter, W., & Achim, A. (2000). Mismatch negativity: Different water in the same river. *Audiology & Neuro-Otology*, *5*(3–4), 111–139.

Pihko, E., Leppasaari, T., & Lyytinen, H. (1995). Brain reacts to occasional changes in duration of elements in a continuous sound. *Neuroreport*, *6*(8), 1215–1218.

Sabri, M. & Campbell, K. B. (2002). The effects of digital filtering on mismatch negativity in wakefulness and slow-wave sleep. *Journal of Sleep Research*, *11*(2), 123–127.

Schroger, E. (1996). The influence of stimulus intensity and inter-stimulus interval on the detection of pitch and loudness changes. *Electroencephalography and Clinical Neurophysiology*, *100*(6), 517–526.

Sinkkonen, J. & Tervaniemi, M. (2000). Towards optimal recording and analysis of the mismatch negativity. *Audiology & Neuro-Otology*, *5*(3–4), 235–246.

Stefanics, G., Haden, G., Huotilainen, M., Balazs, L., Sziller, I., Beke, A., ... Winkler, I. (2007). Auditory temporal grouping in newborn infants. *Psychophysiology*, *44*(5), 697–702. doi: 10.1111/j.1469-8986.2007.00540.x.

Stefanics, G., Haden, G. P., Sziller, I., Balazs, L., Beke, A., & Winkler, I. (2009). Newborn infants process pitch intervals. *Clinical Neurophysiology: Official Journal of the International Federation of Clinical Neurophysiology*, *120*(2), 304–308. doi: 10.1016/j.clinph.2008.11.020.

Tervaniemi, M., Lehtokoski, A., Sinkkonen, J., Virtanen, J., Ilmoniemi, R. J., & Näätänen, R. (1999). Test-retest reliability of mismatch negativity for duration, frequency and intensity changes. *Clinical Neurophysiology: Official Journal of the International Federation of Clinical Neurophysiology*, *110*(8), 1388–1393.

Vigario, R. & Oja, E. (2008). BSS and ICA in neuroinformatics: From current practices to open challenges. *IEEE Reviews in Biomedical Engineering*, *1*, 50–61.

Winkler, I. (2007). Interpreting the mismatch negativity. *Journal of Psychophysiology*, *21*(3–4), 147–163.

www.ingramcontent.com/pod-product-compliance
Lightning Source LLC
Chambersburg PA
CBHW050559190326
41458CB00007B/2107